CMA
Study Guide
2024-2025

Ultimate Exam Blueprint with Advanced Strategies,
All-Inclusive Practice Tests and Audio Lessons to Guarantee
Your First-Time Success as a Certified Medical Assistant

First Try Press

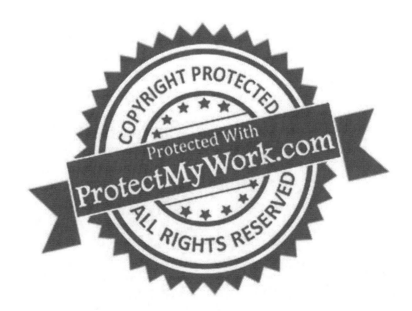

This comprehensive resource is your indispensable partner for conquering the essential principles and abilities necessary for excelling in the CMA examination. Brimming with extensive content, practice exams, and expert guidance, it serves as your route to excellence in one of the healthcare industry's most esteemed certifications.

Table of Contents

Download Your Free Gifts

Please don't forget to leave us a review!

 Download Now

SCAN ME

WELCOME TO THE beginning of your guide to the Certified Medical Assistant (CMA) Exam, an important step on your path to becoming an important member of the healthcare team. Aspiring CMAs like you are about to start on an exciting, hard journey that promises professional development and a rewarding career in the medical industry.

The American Association of Medical Assistants (AAMA) created the CMA Exam, which is a demanding, all-encompassing exam. This exam is intended to confirm that you have the clinical and administrative knowledge required to execute the duties of a medical assistant in the United States.

To become a Certified Medical Assistant, you must first master a variety of abilities, ranging from patient care and procedural aid to administrative chores and office management. As a result, passing the CMA exam ensures that you can maintain the highest professional standards while also contributing to efficient, compassionate patient care.

The exam is divided into four sections, namely general knowledge, administrative knowledge, clinical knowledge, and professional behavior. Each subject covers a variety of topics, ensuring that you are assessed thoroughly on your suitability for the post of CMA.

Let's break down these portions to better grasp what's ahead:

- General: This component evaluates your knowledge of anatomy, medical terminology, pathology, and physiology, as well as patient rapport, communication, and professional demeanor.
- Administrative: Your knowledge of medical reception, patient navigator tasks, practice finances, and medical business procedures will be assessed in this section.
- Clinical: This section of the exam will assess your understanding of asepsis, infection control, aiding with examinations and treatments, patient education, and clinical pharmacology.

- Professional Behavior: This portion assesses your knowledge of ethics, legal elements of medicine, and protective procedures, ensuring that you are equipped to manage challenging settings while remaining professional.

Passing the CMA Exam demonstrates your dedication to the medical assisting field, which can greatly improve your job prospects. By demonstrating your commitment to delivering exceptional patient care, you also showcase your dedication to upholding the professional and ethical standards of the healthcare industry. This can be highly valuable to potential employers.

This guide is intended to completely prepare you for the CMA Exam. We'll go over each exam component in detail in the following chapters, providing clear, concise information, practice questions, and methods to help you pass the exam confidently and effectively.

Remember that becoming a Certified Medical Assistant is way more than getting that certificate. It is about developing a lifelong dedication to learning, improving, and providing the best possible care. Allow this guide to be your beacon as you travel this path, illuminating the way to a successful career as a Certified Medical Assistant.

A Summary of the CMA Exam

As we go deeper into the heart of the CMA Exam, let's look at its key components to ensure you fully understand what's in store. This isn't just a test; it's a critical step in your healthcare career, measuring your readiness to take on substantial responsibilities in a changing medical environment.

The American Association of Medical Assistants organizes the CMA Exam into three basic categories: general, administrative, and clinical. Each category examines different aspects of medical aid, forming a comprehensive assessment of your abilities. Let us go deeper into these categories:

General

This section serves as your medical knowledge foundation. It measures your understanding of fundamental biomedical sciences such as medical terminology, anatomy, physiology, and pathology. It also assesses your knowledge of critical professional factors such as communication, medical legislation, and ethics. The exam confirms you have the core knowledge required for the work of a medical assistant by covering these areas.

Administrative

The administrative components of medical aid are the emphasis of this category. This section assesses your ability to manage the day-to-day operations of a medical office, from scheduling appointments and managing medical records to handling practice finances and insurance processes. The exam confirms your ability to conduct administrative activities efficiently, ensuring the smooth operation of a healthcare environment through this portion.

Clinical

The Clinical category evaluates your hands-on, practical patient care skills. This covers your knowledge of asepsis, infection control, gathering patient information, assisting with examinations and treatments, preparing and giving drugs, and patient education. This section assesses your readiness to assist physicians and provide patient care in a clinical setting.

The CMA Exam covers six broad areas to ensure that you, as a prospective Certified Medical Assistant, can deliver the best level of care to patients and support to physicians. It is a comprehensive examination designed to assess your knowledge and skills while also confirming your dedication to the medical sector.

As we progress through this book, we will go over each topic in depth, giving you in-depth knowledge, tactics, and practice questions. This is your path to passing the CMA Exam and launching a rewarding career in healthcare. The trip may appear difficult, but remember that each step is a step closer to your goal. Stay engaged as we commence on this illuminating journey together.

CHAPTER 1
General Medical Knowledge

WELCOME TO THE first chapter of our guide, where we'll unravel the mysteries of the CMA Exam's General Medical Knowledge section. This chapter will delve into the fundamental scientific ideas that every medical assistant must understand, providing you with the bedrock knowledge required for your work in the healthcare setting.

The General Medical Knowledge area is the foundation of your medical knowledge. This section focuses on the fundamentals of biomedical sciences, which include anatomy, physiology, medical terminology, and pathology. Furthermore, it incorporates crucial professional features like communication, medical law, and ethics, all of which are necessary for developing a well-rounded healthcare professional.

Anatomy and Physiology

Any healthcare worker must understand the human body, the body's systems, and how they work together. This segment examines your understanding of the human body's structure and organs, the many biological systems, their activities, and how they interact. To flourish in this subject, become familiar with fundamental concepts such as cellular structure, body systems (such as the circulatory, neurological, and digestive systems), and their typical function and activities.

As we begin the General Medical Knowledge segment, we start at the heart of healthcare comprehension —Anatomy and Physiology. This crucial section of the CMA exam assesses your understanding of the human body's structure, many functions, and the intricate interplay of its various systems. An effective medical assistant must have a solid understanding of these principles.

Anatomy is the study of the structure of the body, including the bones, muscles, tissues, organs, and interactions. It is about knowing the "where" and "what" of our bodies. From the smallest cellular structures to the largest organ systems, each component has a distinct position and function. This information enables you to accurately follow the physician's directions, deliver drugs correctly, and offer appropriate patient care.

As a medical assistant, you have to understand the major systems of the human body: the muscular, skeletal, endocrine, nervous, respiratory, circulatory, urinary, digestive, and reproductive systems. Each method has its own set of structures and functions that you must properly comprehend. For example, you should understand how the skeletal system offers structural support and protection to the body, as well as the names and locations of the organs and soft tissue structures.

Physiology, on the other hand, investigates the "how"—how our bodies function, how organ systems interact, and how our bodies adapt and respond to changes. The interrelationships between organ systems are complex and dynamic, assisting in the maintenance of balance or homeostasis, which is necessary for survival. Understanding physiology allows you to notice when something isn't working properly, which is an important ability in healthcare.

For example, if you understand the physiology of the cardiovascular system, you'll know that the heart pumps blood, transporting oxygen and nutrients to the body's cells. If this mechanism is disturbed, cells do not obtain what they require, potentially leading to health problems. Your ability to understand such cause-and-effect correlations is an important indicator of your readiness to effectively assist in patient care.

It's worth noting that, while anatomy and physiology are distinct fields of study, they are inextricably linked. A solid study of one improves your understanding of the other. Understanding the structure of the heart (anatomy) will help you comprehend how it pumps blood throughout the body (physiology). Similarly, knowing the shape of the lungs (anatomy) makes comprehending how they exchange gases (physiology) much easier.

By studying anatomy and physiology, you will receive theoretical knowledge and a fundamental understanding that will serve as the foundation for your medical assisting career. It gives you the tools you need to analyze what's going on beneath the skin, identify the underlying cause of a patient's symptoms, and provide appropriate therapeutic support.

Remember, when we explore more into these intriguing issues in the following chapters, that this is the essence of healthcare. Every concept you learn, every link you make, and every system you comprehend moves you closer to becoming an expert medical assistant capable of providing superior patient care. So, keep your curiosity alive, and let's continue exploring the beautiful world of human anatomy and physiology together.

Terminology, Communication, and Ethics in Medicine

As a medical assistant, you will frequently encounter unusual medical jargon. Knowing medical language allows you to interact effectively with patients, insurance companies, and healthcare providers. This exam will test your knowledge of common root words, prefixes, and suffixes used in medicine. You should also be familiar with the abbreviations and symbols that are commonly used in patient records and prescriptions.

Communication:

In the healthcare industry, excellent communication skills are essential. You will frequently act as a liaison between physicians and patients, providing clear and persuasive communication. This section of the exam will assess your abilities to communicate orally and in writing, to recognize nonverbal cues, and to employ therapeutic communication approaches.

Medical Ethics and Law:

To manage healthcare, ethical and legal knowledge is required. As a medical assistant, you will frequently be confronted with situations that necessitate strong judgment based on legal and ethical standards. You must understand patient rights, professional liability, and the legal ramifications of medical documentation. This section of the exam will put your professional and ethical judgment to the test.

The CMA Exam's General Medical Knowledge part is more than just rote memorization—it's about comprehending how these elements interact to develop a comprehensive grasp of healthcare. Remember that while we explore each part of this area in the coming chapters, this knowledge isn't just for passing an exam; it lays the framework for your success as a medical assistant, allowing you to deliver compassionate, informed care to every patient you come into contact with.

Approach this adventure with zeal and curiosity. The more thoroughly you comprehend these ideas, the more skilled and confident you will become as a healthcare professional. Let us embrace the challenge and enjoy each step that brings us closer to becoming outstanding medical assistants as we explore each topic.

Medical Terminology

Medical terminology is a specific language that health professionals use to communicate clearly and effectively. This glossary of medical terminology serves as the foundation of the healthcare communication system, helping you to comprehend, interpret, and convey complex medical information. Mastery of medical terminology is essential for everyday interactions with physicians, other healthcare staff as a medical assistant, and patients.

Medical language can appear complex, even intimidating at first. It does, however, follow a logical structure, breaking down into smaller, more intelligible components such as prefixes, roots, and suffixes. This standardized structure enables a structured, universal method of communicating healthcare-related information, eliminating ambiguity and improving communication clarity.

The heart of medical terms are root words, which usually denote a body part or a condition. They are frequently derived from Greek or Latin roots. For example, the word "cardi" relates to the heart, whereas the term "never" alludes to nerves.

To offer more context or specificity, prefixes are appended to the beginning of root words. For example, "hyper-" denotes excess or above-average, but "hypo-" denotes deficiency or below-average.

Usually appended to the end of the original word to imply a condition, method, or disease. As an example, "it is" refers to inflammation, while "-ectomy" refers to removal or excision.

Many medical terminologies can be deciphered by combining these components. For example, the word "carditis" can be broken down into "cardi-" (heart) and "-it is" (inflammation), indicating that the heart is inflamed. Similarly, the word "neurology" is made up of the words "near-" (nerve) and "-ology" (study of), denoting the breakdown of nerves.

Understanding commonly used medical abbreviations, in addition to these components, is critical to your medical terminology knowledge. Abbreviations assist in expressing information quickly and efficiently in the fast-paced medical environment. Be cautious, however, because certain abbreviations might have numerous meanings. To ensure the right interpretation, always consider the context.

Understanding medical language assists you in doing your job as a medical assistant more efficiently. It facilitates the interpretation of physician's notes, the transcription of medical records, the explanation of procedures to patients, and communication with other healthcare professionals. More importantly, it aids in the reduction of misunderstandings, which is critical in patient safety.

The CMA Exam examines your grasp of medical language, ensuring that you can navigate the healthcare environment successfully. As you learn more about medical terminology, you'll discover that it broadens your comprehension and equips you to make a more significant contribution to patient care.

While studying medical terminology may appear daunting, keep in mind that it is all about breaking down complex concepts into simpler components. You will grow more comfortable and proficient with constant practice and study. Stay committed, and you will familiarize these formerly new terms in no time.

Keep in mind that you are learning the language of your profession—a language that will allow you to interact with, comprehend, and contribute to the world of healthcare. So, keep that spark of interest alive, and let's continue to delve into this intriguing element of your medical assistant education.

Pathology

The study of diseases is referred to as pathology. It discusses disease causes, consequences on the body, symptoms, and the body's response to sickness. Understanding pathology allows you to foresee probable problems, grasp a physician's diagnosis, and explain difficult situations to patients in an understandable manner. This component of your general medical knowledge is critical to providing the best possible treatment to patients.

As we continue our journey through the medical environment, we reach a critical point: Pathology and Disease Processes. The nature and causes of diseases, their consequences on the body, and the body's responses to these disorders are all covered in this section of your CMA Exam.

Pathology knowledge is vital for a medical assistant since it allows for proper interpretation of symptoms, good communication with other healthcare professionals, and meaningful support for patient care.

Diseases can result from several factors, such as genetic anomalies, infections, environmental impacts, lifestyle choices, and age. Pathology is concerned with how these factors show as illnesses.

Consider inflammation, which is a common reaction to injury or infection. Recognizing the cardinal indications of inflammation—heat, redness, swelling, pain, and loss of function—can aid in the detection of an inflammatory illness. Similarly, recognizing the usual stages of infection—from incubation through disease resolution—can help in the management of infectious disorders.

Pathology also includes the examination of tissues and cells. Histopathology, for example, investigates the microscopic alterations that diseases induce in bodily tissues, and it is crucial in disease detection. While you may not administer these tests as a medical assistant, learning the fundamentals can help you better serve the healthcare team.

Pathology also encompasses the study of systemic diseases, which are ailments that affect the entire body, such as diabetes or hypertension. Understanding the pathophysiology of these diseases—how they impair normal biological functions—will improve your capacity to aid in patient treatment and education. The pathology component of the CMA Exam assesses your capacity to appreciate these disease processes, cultivating an astute medical assistant capable of interpreting clinical symptoms, comprehending diagnostic tests, and facilitating appropriate treatment methods.

As we go deeper into pathology, keep in mind that knowing these disease processes is about training you to better support your patients. It prepares you to recognize the potential consequences of symptoms, empathize with the patient's situation, and present complex health facts in a way that patients can understand.

Pathology may appear difficult to learn, but it is all about piecing together the jigsaw of the human body's response to disease. Keep asking questions, and the complicated tapestry of disease processes will eventually unfold in front of you.

Remember that this knowledge enables you to make a major benefit to patient care. So, keep your curiosity alive, and join us as we continue our exploration of the intriguing realm of pathology and disease processes.

Pharmacology and Medication Administration

The science of drugs is called pharmacology. It investigates how drugs interact with the biological systems of the body, influencing physiological functioning. It is the art of healing, comforting, and, in many cases, life-saving measures. As a medical assistant, you'll be dealing with pharmaceuticals regularly, so understanding pharmacology is both a responsibility and a requirement.

We evaluate various criteria when researching a drug. These include the generic and brand names of the medicine, its therapeutic class, the problems it is used to treat, and its mechanism of action (how it creates its therapeutic effect). Understanding a drug's mode of administration, dose forms, common adverse effects, and potential drug interactions is also critical for pharmaceutical safety.

The drug life cycle, also known as pharmacokinetics, is a fundamental topic in pharmacology. It describes the process by which a medication is absorbed, distributed, metabolized, and eventually removed from the body. These dynamics influence medicine dosage and timing to guarantee the best therapeutic outcome.

Pharmacodynamics, or the study of how medications affect the body, is also critical. It investigates the drug-receptor interaction and how it affects cell activity. Pharmacodynamics predicts a drug's therapeutic and unfavorable effects, facilitating the selection of the best treatment for a patient.

Pharmacology also includes drug classification. Drugs are frequently classified according to their therapeutic impact, such as analgesics for pain alleviation, antihypertensives for high blood pressure control, or antibiotics for treating bacterial infections. Understanding these classifications allows you to understand the reason for a patient's pharmaceutical regimen. Furthermore, pharmacology research emphasizes the significance of the "Five Rights" of pharmaceutical administration: the right patient, the right drug, the right dose, the right route, and the right time. Following these principles is critical in reducing pharmaceutical errors and protecting patient health.

Your job in pharmacology as a medical assistant goes beyond simply understanding medicines. It entails teaching patients about their prescriptions, monitoring for side effects, and advocating for patient safety. These assignments are built on your pharmacology knowledge, which promotes improved patient outcomes.

The pharmacology component of the CMA Exam tests your understanding of these topics, preparing you to handle drugs properly and confidently. Pharmacology may appear to be a big and confusing field, but it is all about getting to know these therapeutic instruments, knowing their advantages and disadvantages, and optimizing their use for patient benefit.

Remember that each medication you learn, each drug interaction you comprehend, and each side effect you notice is a step closer to becoming an outstanding medical assistant. It equips you to help provide effective, safe, and patient-centered care.

So, let us embrace this learning adventure, comprehend the tremendous impact of pharmacology, and discover your important position in medication management. Your interest in pharmacology is more than simply an academic pursuit; it is a road that will lead you closer to becoming a vital member of the healthcare team.

Examples of Common Drugs in Medical Practice

1. Analgesics (Pain Relievers):
   o Acetaminophen (Tylenol)
   o Ibuprofen (Advil, Motrin)
   o Naproxen (Aleve)
   o Morphine
   o Oxycodone (OxyContin)
2. Antibiotics:
   o Penicillin

- o   Amoxicillin
- o   Ciprofloxacin (Cipro)
- o   Azithromycin (Zithromax)
- o   Doxycycline (Vibramycin)
3. Antidepressants:
    - o   Sertraline (Zoloft)
    - o   Fluoxetine (Prozac)
    - o   Escitalopram (Lexapro)
    - o   Citalopram (Celexa)
    - o   Venlafaxine (Effexor)
4. Antihypertensives (Blood Pressure Medications):
    - o   Amlodipine (Norvasc)
    - o   Lisinopril (Prinivil, Zestril)
    - o   Metoprolol (Lopressor)
    - o   Losartan (Cozaar)
    - o   Hydrochlorothiazide (HCTZ)
5. Antidiabetic Medications:
    - o   Metformin (Glucophage)
    - o   Insulin (various types)
    - o   Glipizide (Glucotrol)
    - o   Sitagliptin (Januvia)
    - o   Liraglutide (Victoza)
6. Anticoagulants (Blood Thinners):
    - o   Warfarin (Coumadin)
    - o   Rivaroxaban (Xarelto)
    - o   Apixaban (Eliquis)
    - o   Dabigatran (Pradaxa)
7. Antihistamines (Allergy Medications):
    - o   Loratadine (Claritin)
    - o   Cetirizine (Zyrtec)
    - o   Diphenhydramine (Benadryl)
    - o   Fexofenadine (Allegra)

8. Antipsychotics:
   o Risperidone (Risperdal)
   o Quetiapine (Seroquel)
   o Olanzapine (Zyprexa)
   o Aripiprazole (Abilify)
   o Haloperidol (Haldol)

9. Bronchodilators (Respiratory Medications):
   o Albuterol (Proventil, Ventolin)
   o Ipratropium (Atrovent)
   o Salmeterol (Serevent)
   o Budesonide/Formoterol (Symbicort)

10. Antacids and Gastrointestinal Medications:
    o Ranitidine (Zantac)
    o Omeprazole (Prilosec)
    o Metoclopramide (Reglan)
    o Loperamide (Imodium)

11. Thyroid Medications:
    o Levothyroxine (Synthroid)
    o Liothyronine (Cytomel)
    o Thyroid desiccated (Armour Thyroid)

12. Vaccines:
    o Influenza vaccine
    o MMR vaccine (Measles, Mumps, Rubella)
    o Hepatitis B vaccine
    o COVID-19 vaccines (e.g., Pfizer-BioNTech, Moderna, Johnson & Johnson)

Pharmacokinetics

Pharmacokinetics is the study of distribution, medication absorption, excretion from the body, and metabolism. Pharmacokinetics knowledge improves treatment and reduces side effects. For instance, people with end-stage liver illness should utilize medications that are metabolized in the liver with extreme caution. Similar to how someone having an intense seizure is treated with a suppository rather than an oral drug because they are unable to swallow.

All pharmaceuticals must be stored properly, and humidity, temperature, and light exposure should all be considered. Finally, there are regulations governing the disposal of medications, and all facilities are required to provide safe ways to get rid of sharps and needles.

Packaging and Form

There are many different ways to take medications, including tablets, vials, suppositories, gels, ointments, and transdermal patches. The majority of parenteral medications for injection are offered in premixed vials, although sometimes preparation is necessary. The methods for administering medications and the formulae that are accessible must be known by medical assistants:

Multidose vials are used to provide the medication to numerous people, however extreme caution must be exercised to prevent contamination of the remaining medication during withdrawal. Before inserting the needle, the plastic or rubber stopper should be frequently cleaned with alcohol wipes.

Typically, ampoules hold just enough medication for a single dose. The vial is typically scored at the neck to make it simple to break and draw up the solution using a needle and syringe.

Unit doses are single, prepared dosages of injectable or oral medications. Despite being hermetically sealed, once they are opened, the medication must be consumed.

The premixed, ready-to-inject cartridge-needle units come in vials. Some have needles built inside the vial.

In order to use many drugs, they must first be reconstituted in saline or water. These medications are typically provided in powder form. These sealed, single-dose vials are simple to use.

Prescriptions and Refills

You will be responsible for placing new drug orders and approving refills for several chronic patients as a member of a clinic. Refills must adhere to tight guidelines, and documentation is mandatory for all prescription medications. You will need to order and prescribe drugs in accordance with the clinic's policies.

Regulations

All prescription medications are governed by the US Food and Drug Administration, which medical assistants should be informed of. Over-the-counter products are subject to less strict regulation. The Drug Enforcement Agency (DEA) is a federal regulatory organization that establishes guidelines for issuing, ordering, replenishing, storing, and recording all banned narcotics. The majority of banned substances are highly susceptible to abuse and physical dependence. Nowadays, computerized prescriptions are issued in the vast majority of cases. Both written and digital prescriptions for oral medications are available. It's crucial to understand that only a particular number of medications can be distributed in a given period of time. The frequency of refills is likewise constrained in practice. A qualified doctor with a current DEA number must be involved if the patient requests a refill of a controlled substance.

Preparation and Administration

Preparing and giving drugs to patients is one of the tasks that medical assistants will perform frequently. Although it may seem insignificant, it is crucial that you pay attention and take your time while performing these tasks. Always get clarification from a senior individual if an order is difficult to read, imprecise, or ambiguous. Never ask someone else to prepare or take your drugs for you. Ask the patient once more whether they have any allergies before giving them the medication.

Always check your work twice.

Six Rights of Medication Administration

The following six rights of medicine administration have been created to ensure pharmaceutical safety and should be followed at all times.

1. The right patient: Verify the patient's entire name and birthday before administering the drug.
2. The right drug: Ensure that you are giving the appropriate medication. Finally, make sure it is the proper drug before you administer it by double-checking when you pick up the order.

3. The right time: Always check with the patient to see if it's time for them to take their prescription.

4. The right dose: Always make sure the dosage matches what was specified in the order. Verify again with the ordering healthcare professional.

5. The right route: Always confirm that the drug will be administered according to the order's specified method of administration.

6. The right documentation: Document every aspect of the drug administration, including the date, time, drug name, dosage, and method of administration, in the patient's medical records. You should also note whether the drug was tolerated.

Measurements

You occasionally might have to provide a liquid drug to a patient, and you'll need to be familiar with the measurements. A cc is equivalent to a ml. Five milliliters (5 ml) make up a teaspoon (abb tsp), while 15 ml make up a tablespoon. Basic math skills are required for conversion. For instance, if the patient needs two teaspoons, this translates to 2 x 5 ml, or 10 ml.

Another illustration: How much medication would a patient take in total over the course of five days if he takes one tablespoon twice daily?

First off, a tablespoon contains 15 ml.

He takes it twice daily, which works out to 30 ml (2 x 15 ml). He uses it for five days, thus the total amount is 30 x 5 = 150 ml.

Administration Routes

The various methods of medicine administration must be known by medical assistants.

- Oral medications (capsules, liquids, pills)
- Sublingual or buccal (tablets absorbed under the tongue or in the cheek)
- Transdermal (medications absorbed through the skin via a patch or cream)
- Mucosal absorption medications (rectal or vaginal suppositories)

- Respiratory inhalers (nebulized medications)
- Parenteral (subcutaneous, SQ, intravenous, IV, or intramuscular IM injections)
- Intraosseous (meds delivered into the medullary space of a bone)
- Intradermal (injected between dermal layers of the skin)

Parenteral

In addition to intravenous injection, injectable drugs may also be given subcutaneously (into the subcutaneous fat), or intramuscularly (into a large muscle).

These drugs frequently cannot be taken by mouth since doing so might cause them to lose their effectiveness or cause them to degrade in the stomach.

The subcutaneous fat is injected with a subcutaneous (SQ) needle. Insulin is a prime illustration.

IM injections are administered in the deltoid, ventrogluteal, or thigh. Injections into the IM are frequently used to give steroids.

The intradermal injection is given directly below the surface of the skin. When testing for tuberculosis, the PPD intradermal test is usually employed.

IM Injections

Applied to both adults and kids

The sites for adults are the deltoid, ventrogluteal, or thigh.

For pediatrics, the lateral thigh is preferable.

Adults should only have a maximum volume of 2 ml in their upper arm and 5 ml in their thigh.

Children should only have a maximum volume of 2 ml, and newborns should get less than 0.5 ml.

Needle length and gauge:

1. The point of injection determines the length and gauge of the needle. A large gauge and a longer length are needed for deep injections. Adults can safely administer an IM injection using a 20–23 gauge needle.
2. The gauge for intradermal injections should be 30–31, and their length should not exceed 0.5 inches.
3. Subcutaneous injections require needles with gauges of 25–27 and lengths of less than 0.5 inches.

Administering the medication:

1. Before administering medicines, follow the six rights of medication administration
2. Always put on gloves and clean the site of injection with an alcohol wipe or chlorhexidine
3. Always aspirate before administering an intramuscular injection to make sure you have not injected into a blood vessel
4. Massage is permitted following IM drug delivery
5. Dispose of the needle and syringe in accordance with the facility's rules

Medication Formula

Single-unit dosages, multidose vials, prefilled cartridge needle units, and ampules are just a few of the several forms that injectable drugs that can be found.

Every clinic or healthcare facility has policies in place regarding the proper handling and disposal of sharp objects, such as needles and syringes. To avoid harm or mistakes, you must adhere to these rules.

For the needle, scalpel, and syringe disposal, the facility should generally have a labeled sharps container. Today, many needles and syringes have built-in safety features to guard against needle sticks, protecting both patients and staff.

Other Routes

The different medicine administration methods that you will need to be knowledgeable about as a medical assistant are included in this list.

Oral—comprises pills, elixirs, syrups, and capsules. Some of these drugs, such as nitroglycerin for chest pain, may not be entirely absorbed from the stomach and may need to be given sublingually.

Inhalers—Nebulizers, dry powder inhalers, and meter dosage inhalers are all types of inhalers that are available. They can also be given via a mask or nasal cannula along with oxygen. The inhaler's medicine delivery to the airway causes an immediate effect.

Topicals—Ointments, creams, gels, and pledgets are examples of topicals. Typically, these topicals are given to healthy skin. To improve the medication's absorption into the systemic circulation, an occlusive bandage may occasionally be placed over it. Transdermal patches are frequently used to administer hormones like estrogen and painkillers like fentanyl.

Delivering drops to the eye, nose, or ears is referred to as installation. To treat an allergy, or illness, or to ease discomfort, the drops may be utilized. The patient must be positioned properly to ensure that the drops are instilled and will work.

Vaginal—Medications may occasionally be inserted in the vagina. These drugs, which come in the form of pills, suppositories, or lotions, are mostly used as contraceptives or to treat infections. The absorption happens quickly due to the vagina's high blood flow.

Rectal—Like the vagina, the rectum contains a sizable mucosal surface that facilitates medication absorption. Thus, medications like NSAIDs, antiemetics, antiseizure medications, and opioids are frequently administered as suppositories. When a person has a severe swallowing problem, the rectal route is a very effective medicine delivery strategy.

Other Topics

CMAs will likely be involved in administering vaccines to both adults and children in addition to preparing and administering drugs. So, it is likely that the medical assistant will need to complete additional coursework and training to administer immunizations and avoid difficulties. There are vaccines available for polio, varicella, HPV, zoster, and pneumonia in addition to the annual flu shot. These vaccinations are often given according to a schedule, and the majority call for many doses spaced out over a few months. Additionally, each vaccine has particular storage needs. The CDC does offer a vaccine information sheet that describes the vaccine's dangers and advantages. Before giving the vaccine, patients must receive the vaccine information statement (VIS).

Documentation must be kept after each vaccination and must include the date, lot number, patient's name, address, time, and the person's name who gave the shot. The injection site and the patient's tolerance should also be mentioned.

Administration Documentation

As soon as meds are administered, medical assistants should note it in the patient's chart. Time, date, medicine name, dose, frequency, route, and, if applicable, location of administration should all be included in the paperwork. It is important to note how the drug affected the patient.

Even if the patient doesn't experience any side effects, a pharmaceutical error, such as giving the wrong dose, the wrong patient, or the wrong substance, must be recorded in the patient's documentation. Ensuring that this never occurs again is crucial.

Summary

- General Medical Knowledge is the foundation for a medical assistant's work in healthcare.
- It covers anatomy, physiology, medical terminology, pathology, communication, medical ethics, and law.
- Understanding anatomy and physiology is crucial for comprehending the functions and structure of the human body.

- Medical terminology involves root words, prefixes, and suffixes used in healthcare communication.

- Pathology explores the causes, effects, and responses to diseases, aiding in patient care.

- Pharmacology is vital for understanding drugs, their effects, and safe administration.

- Learning these subjects equips you to provide better patient care and effectiveness in healthcare.

- Medication Knowledge: CMAs should have a strong understanding of common medications, including their generic and brand names, common abbreviations, and administration methods.

- Medication Safety: Ensuring patient safety is paramount. CMAs must adhere to the "Six Rights of Medication Administration" to guarantee the right patient, medication, route, timing, dosage, and proper documentation.

- Pharmacokinetics: Understanding how drugs are absorbed, distributed, metabolized, and excreted in the body is important for tailoring medication administration.

- Storage and Disposal: Properly storing medications and adhering to regulations for disposal, especially sharps disposal, are critical.

- Administration Methods: CMAs need to be knowledgeable about various medication administration routes, including injections (intramuscular, intradermal, subcutaneous), oral medications, inhalers, topical applications, and more.

- Vaccinations: Familiarity with vaccine administration, schedules, storage requirements, and documentation is essential.

- Regulations: Awareness of FDA and DEA regulations, particularly for controlled substances, is necessary.

- Measurement Skills: Proficiency in measurement units for liquid medications, including conversions, is important.

- Documentation: Accurate and comprehensive documentation of medication administration, including date, time, medication specifics, and patient response, is crucial.

CHAPTER 2

Administrative Work

WE CAN'T IGNORE the importance of administrative components in healthcare as we delve into the multifaceted work of a Certified Medical Assistant (CMA). This section of the CMA Exam assesses your knowledge of administrative responsibilities, highlighting the importance of skills other than patient care. These include everything from organizing medical records to assisting with insurance processes and helping the seamless operation of a healthcare facility.

The first image that comes to mind when you think of a medical assistant is one of a healthcare practitioner assisting in clinical operations. While this is an important aspect of the job, a medical assistant is also the backbone of administrative operations in healthcare facilities.

Medical assistants are the facility's front-line representatives. They greet patients, schedule appointments, answer phones, and run the front desk. Patients' perceptions of the healthcare institution can be strongly influenced by their professionalism, communication skills, and efficiency.

The major administrative function of a medical assistant is to manage patient records. This entails accurately recording and updating patient information, as well as preserving these records' confidentiality and security. Given their ubiquitous use in modern healthcare institutions, knowledge of Electronic Health Records (EHRs) systems is frequently required.

Medical assistants are very important in the insurance process. They verify/confirm the insurance information and submit claims, and they may also be in charge of billing and coding. This necessitates a thorough awareness of health insurance regulations, billing methods, and diagnostic and procedure codes.

In addition to these duties, medical assistants do a variety of administrative activities such as ordering and doing inventory of the medical supplies, handling communications, as well as even working with the public relations and marketing activities of the healthcare center.

A CMA's administrative duty is distinguished by its role as a liaison. They act as a bridge between the healthcare team and the patient, the patient and their insurance provider, or even different members of the healthcare team. This requires good communication skills as well as a patient-centered approach.

Why are administrative tasks so important in healthcare? This is due to two factors. First and foremost, efficient administrative processes are vital to the smooth and effective administration of a healthcare facility. They shorten wait times, avoid schedule conflicts, and improve the patient experience. Second, they free up some healthcare provider duties to focus on their priorities and responsibility: patient care. Medical assistants free providers from administrative duties, prolonging their time with patients, thereby improving care quality.

The Administrative Aspects section of the CMA exam will challenge what you learned and your responsibilities and principles. It's not only a matter of memorizing procedures or learning software. It is about having knowledge on the "why" of each task. As a result, the significance of your role is appreciated and how you may contribute to a pleasant patient experience is comprehended.

Remember that every patient encounter, correctly updated record, and effectively submitted insurance claim contribute to patient happiness and excellent care. As a medical assistant, you help healthcare practitioners and improve patient care in ways that aren't often obvious but are crucial.

So, let's take a closer look at the administrative parts of working as a medical assistant. It delves into the mechanisms that keep a healthcare institution functioning properly and your participation in them. It is about determining how you can have a substantial impact on patient care outside of the clinical context.

Medical Reception

Let's take a look at one of the most important positions in the administrative realm of a medical assistant's responsibilities: Medical Reception. The medical receptionist frequently takes the lead for the entire patient visit. The receptionist's eyes and gestures frequently define the healthcare facility's first and last impression.

A medical receptionist's job is more than just welcoming patients and answering phones; it requires a careful balance of interpersonal skills, organization, and knowledge of medical terminologies and protocols. The medical receptionist is the face of the healthcare center, the initial point of contact, and an administrative powerhouse all at the same time.

Scheduling patient appointments is a critical function of the medical receptionist. Managing a complex schedule, addressing patient demands, and adjusting for unanticipated events, such as emergencies or cancellations, are all part of the job. In the healthcare facility, efficient scheduling saves the provider's time, minimizes the wait times of patients, and promotes a more efficient workflow.

Aside from scheduling, the receptionist is responsible for the registration of patients and keeping their records up to date. This includes gathering relevant personal and insurance information from patients and making sure that it is input accurately into the system. When a patient database is well-organized, it provides better patient care, billing and insurance processes, and communication.

Notably, the medical receptionist is in charge of communication within the hospital. Receiving and making phone calls, managing correspondence, and liaising between patients and healthcare professionals are all part of the job. Each communication touchpoint represents a chance to provide exceptional service while also fostering a positive patient environment.

Medical receptionists frequently have various behind-the-scenes obligations in addition to their patient-facing roles. They handle the reception area, keep office supplies in order, and may assist with basic financial responsibilities like co-pay collection or billing inquiries. A clean, well-organized welcome area improves patient comfort and confidence in the healthcare institution, while efficient resource management helps the overall efficiency of the facility.

Every encounter and activity you perform as a medical receptionist has an impact. Your words calm a nervous patient; your organizational skills make a healthcare provider's schedule better, and your efficiency ups the institution's general performance.

The CMA Exam's Medical Reception segment will assess your ability to accomplish these duties. It will put your knowledge of administrative procedures, communication skills, and healthcare systems to the test. It is about demonstrating your readiness to serve as the face of the healthcare facility, the initial point of contact in a patient's care journey.

But keep in mind that being a medical receptionist entails more than just passing an exam. It's about recognizing how you can improve a patient's experience. It's about realizing how important your administrative position is to patient care.

Let us recall the power we have as we investigate the job of a medical receptionist. The smile we give, the reassuring phrase, and the efficient action we take move us a step closer to becoming not only a medical receptionist but also a key contributor to patient care.

Patient Navigator/Advocate

Before we get into the intricacies of the function of a patient Navigator/Advocate, it's important to understand the significance of this position. In healthcare, a patient's path is frequently plagued with confusion and worry. Patients may feel lost and overwhelmed as they navigate the maze of medical terminology, insurance processes, and several specialist appointments.

This is when a Patient Navigator/Advocate comes in handy. As a Certified Medical Assistant (CMA), you will be able to assist patients beyond acute medical care, making a big difference in their health-care journey. Let us explore this critical job and learn what it takes to be a true patient navigator and advocate.

Understanding the Role

A CMA wears multiple hats in today's healthcare system. One of the most important is their role as patient navigator or advocate. As a lighthouse of support and advice, this role focuses on navigating patients through the intricate healthcare web. A patient navigator/advocate makes sure that patients receive essential medical care while also understanding and navigating the complexities of the health-care system.

Bridging the Gap

A Patient Navigator/Advocate's function is to serve as a liaison between the healthcare system and the patient. As a CMA, you are required to lead patients through the maze of healthcare, acting as a guidepost for medical language, procedures, and insurance systems. You take on the role of a vital liaison, coordinating care and explaining the difficulties.

Coordination of Care

Care coordination is an important part of being a Patient Navigator/Advocate. As a CMA, you will be responsible for scheduling appointments, following up with specialists, ensuring timely medical tests, and monitoring treatment regimens. This component needs a thorough awareness of the healthcare system as well as high-level organization skills. But, more crucially, it necessitates understanding and compassion for the sufferers.

Communication—the Key

The heart of patient advocacy is effective communication. Your position as a Patient Navigator/Advocate entails describing medical words, insurance claims, and procedures in a way that patients can understand. This de-mystification of medical jargon can provide comfort to patients, decreasing stress and empowering them to make educated health decisions.

Support Beyond Medical Care

A Patient Navigator/Advocate's assistance frequently extends beyond medical care. You could be aiding patients with insurance paperwork, researching financial assistance possibilities, or offering emotional support. Your job may vary, but the goal remains the same: to make a patient's trip through healthcare as seamless and stress-free as possible.

Getting Ready for the CMA Exam

The Patient Navigator/Advocate section of the CMA exam will examine your grasp of these tasks. It will assess your communication skills, your capacity to coordinate treatment, your grasp of medical and insurance processes, and your empathy and commitment to patient welfare.

However, keep in mind that your position as a Patient Navigator/Advocate is more than just passing an exam. It is all about creating a real difference and impact on healthcare experience of a patient. It's about metaphorically—and sometimes, literally—holding a patient's hand as they travel the perilous path of healthcare.

What Really Is the Heart of Patient Advocacy

Being a Patient Navigator/Advocate means accepting that you play an important role in patient care. You are the tour guide, comforter, organizer, and interpreter. You play a role in shaping the patient's experience and perception of healthcare.

Remember the underlying theme as we go deeper into the responsibilities of a Patient Navigator/Advocate: it's all about the patient. It's about their wants, their comfort, and their comprehension. It is about making healthcare less intimidating and more empathetic. The goal is to make a difference in a patient's life, one at a time.

Medical Business Practices

Healthcare extends much beyond the acute medical care given to patients. Medical Business Practices are an important, if less visible, feature at the junction of healthcare and business. Although not having direct involvement in patient care, these practices are essential to the proper administration of a healthcare institution, making sure that medical professionals provide their patients with timely and effective care.

Your position as a Certified Medical Assistant (CMA) extends into these administrative areas, making you a valued tool in the healthcare business. This section digs into the significance, components, and application of Medical Business Practices to equip CMAs with the right knowledge of handling the business side of healthcare.

The Crossroad of Medicine and Business

Medical Business Practices exist at the crossroads of healthcare and administration. While healthcare professionals focus on providing high-quality medical care, sound business procedures must also be taken into account. These procedures guarantee that healthcare facilities run smoothly, increasing patient care and the institution's financial health.

Understanding Medical Business Practices as a Certified Medical Assistant (CMA) is critical for properly managing the non-clinical aspects of a healthcare facility.

Why Medical Business Practices Are Important

The crux of Medical Business Practices is their significance in ensuring the smooth operation of healthcare organizations. Healthcare institutions may streamline their procedures, improve patient happiness, and assure optimal resource usage by employing business principles. This includes responsibilities like organizing patient appointments, keeping medical records, billing, and insurance processing, all of which are critical in a healthcare setting.

Scheduling and Organization

Scheduling and organizing are two of the initial elements of good medical business procedures. A well-organized system is essential for properly operating a healthcare institution, from tracking patient appointments to arranging staff schedules. It not only increases worker productivity but also assures that patients receive care on schedule.

Medical Records Administration

Accurate and effective medical record administration is the foundation of any healthcare facility. Medical records provide crucial patient information that is required for providing optimal healthcare. Managing effective records means ensuring that these facts are available when needed and improves the quality of care provided.

Billing and Insurance Administration

Another critical part of medical business operations is navigating the realm of healthcare finance, including insurance and billing processing. Being equipped with these processes allows a more pleasant patient experience and the financial stability of the healthcare facility.

Laws and Compliance

The healthcare industry is regulated highly. It has many compliance requirements. Compliance with laws and regulations safeguards both the institution and the patient. It guarantees patient privacy, healthcare quality, and ethical practice. As a result, understanding healthcare rules and regulations is critical to medical business practices.

Exam Preparation for the CMA

The CMA exam's Medical Business Practices section examines your knowledge in these areas. It assesses your ability to schedule, organize, keep records, bill, handle insurance, and comply with the law. With a good grasp of these practices, you can make a contribution substantial to the efficient operation of any healthcare facility.

CMA's Role in Medical Business Practices

As a CMA, you play an important role in Medical Business Practices. You make certain that the business side of healthcare operates efficiently, allowing doctors to focus on providing exceptional patient care. You can contribute through your work to the patient experience, the financial viability of the institution, and healthcare quality, making you a vital asset in the healthcare industry.

Remember that when we go into more detail about the Medical Business Practices, the goal is not simply to pass an exam, but to become well-equipped to efficiently manage the non-clinical components of a healthcare facility. It's about keeping the wheels of healthcare spinning smoothly and, as a result, helping to provide the best possible patient care.

Patient Medical Records

The creation and management of patient medical records are critical to the healthcare delivery system. The records herein are way more than just being a compilation of medical histories and treatment plans; they are critical in maintaining patient care continuity and quality.

A well-managed medical record is a goldmine of patient data that enables healthcare practitioners to make well-informed choices and provide personalized treatment. Understanding how to create patient medical records is critical as a Certified Medical Assistant (CMA).

The Crucial Role of Medical Records

The primary source of information for healthcare practitioners is a patient's medical record, containing pieces of information regarding the patient's diagnostic tests, medical history, progress notes, treatment plans, and other important details. This comprehensive document makes medical care more unified, effective, and personalized.

Establishing Medical Records: The Initial Step

In creating a medical record, it begins with the initial visit of a patient to the healthcare practitioner. During this visit, fundamental pieces of information are attained: the patient's personal info, reason, and medical history. The medical record is constructed on this foundation, and its correctness is critical for good healthcare delivery.

Essential Medical Information Inclusion

Following the initial data gathering, the medical record must be populated with increasingly particular medical information. This includes any diagnoses, medications administered, surgery history, allergies, immunizations, and any other pertinent healthcare information. Every visit that ensues, including treatment plan and diagnosis, is added to this record, resulting in a detailed narrative of the patient's medical journey.

Maintaining Confidentiality and Ensuring Compliance

When managing patient medical records, CMAs must rigorously follow the Health Insurance Portability and Accountability Act (HIPAA) rules. This law protects patient information and establishes stringent rules for the handling of medical records. A CMA must guarantee that these standards are followed to protect the patient's privacy and the integrity of the healthcare facility.

Electronic Health Records (EHRs): The Role of Technology

In today's digital age, most healthcare facilities have transitioned from using paper for records to Electronic Health Records (EHRs). These digital records make patient information more accessible, improve communication among healthcare practitioners, and allow for more effective patient care management. Understanding how EHR systems work is essential for a CMA to successfully manage patient records.

The Foundations of Quality Healthcare

It is impossible to overstate the significance of properly establishing and managing patient medical records. These records are critical in providing patients with effective, personalized care. They improve healthcare provider communication and give vital data quality improvement activities and research.

As a CMA, your role in creating and keeping these records is critical to providing great healthcare. As we proceed, keep in mind that the complexities of medical records administration extend beyond passing an exam. It is about learning skills that will improve patient care, streamline healthcare processes, and make a significant contribution to the healthcare delivery system.

Scheduling Appointments and Practice

As a Certified Medical Assistant (CMA), your responsibilities extend beyond patient care and into administrative duties. Appointment scheduling and practice financial management are two such critical factors. A harmonious appointment system ensures that patients move smoothly and efficiently. Hence, having to understand practice finances is critical to the medical practice's economic health and viability. This section delves into these interrelated responsibilities in depth.

The Art of Managing Schedules

Appointment scheduling is frequently compared to a balancing act. CMAs must ensure a smooth flow of patients while not overbooking or underbooking the time of healthcare providers. The goal is to shorten patient wait times while allowing healthcare practitioners adequate time to offer quality care to each patient.

An efficient scheduling system takes into account the cause of the visit, predicting the time required for various sorts of appointments. Periodic follow-ups, new patient visits, and emergencies necessitate more time. Furthermore, CMAs should take into account the healthcare provider's availability and preferences.

With the rise of digital solutions comes electronic appointment scheduling becoming a norm. It benefits patients and improves the efficiency of healthcare practices. Understanding how such systems work is a necessary ability for CMAs.

An Overview of Managing Practice Finances

Managing practice finances, on the other hand, entails several responsibilities, including but not limited to insurance claims, billing, financial reporting, and budgeting. A good grasp of these financial issues enables a medical practice to sustain itself, guaranteeing that patient treatment can continue.

As a CMA, you could be responsible for preparing patient bills and receiving payments. Understanding the fundamentals of medical coding and billing is required for this work. Accurate billing guarantees that the practice is fairly compensated for the services rendered.

Another critical aspect is the handling of insurance claims. CMAs must grasp the many types of insurance policies, how to follow up on unpaid claims, and the claims filing procedure. Having understood this process by heart ensures prompt recompense and avoids financial strain on the practice.

Budgeting and financial reporting are vital for a CMA to grasp, even if they are often handled by practice managers or financial officers. CMAs can contribute to financial conversations and make informed judgments about practice operations if they have a basic comprehension of these procedures.

The Reciprocity Between Scheduling and Finances

At first look, scheduling and finance may appear to be separate concepts. They are, nonetheless, inextricably intertwined. Effective scheduling makes the best use of resources, increasing the financial efficiency of the practice. For example, proper scheduling can dramatically improve a practice's financial health by reducing no-shows and cancellations.

CMAs: The Key Pillars of an Efficient Practice

Finally, CMAs are critical in sustaining the administrative synchronization of a healthcare practice. The ability to efficiently arrange appointments and comprehend practice finances is critical to your work as a CMA.

While these activities may appear onerous at first, with time and practice, they will become second nature to you. As a CMA, your participation in these administrative aspects makes you an important member of the healthcare team, guaranteeing a seamless operation while focusing on what is most important—patient care.

Summary

General Administrative Duties:

- Medical assistants have a vital role in healthcare administration, beyond clinical tasks.

- They are front-line representatives, managing patient interactions, scheduling, and more.
- Efficient administrative processes are essential for smooth healthcare facility operations.
- Managing Patient Records:
- Medical assistants play a significant role in managing patient records and ensuring accuracy and confidentiality.
- Knowledge of Electronic Health Records (EHRs) is often required in modern healthcare.

Insurance Processes:

- Medical assistants are involved in insurance processes, including verification, claims submission, billing, and coding.
- They need a deep understanding of health insurance regulations and codes.

Various Administrative Activities:

- Medical assistants handle inventory management, and communications, and may engage in marketing and public relations.
- They act as liaisons between patients, healthcare teams, and insurance providers, requiring strong communication skills.

Importance of Administrative Tasks:

- Efficient administrative processes improve the patient experience and provide extra time for healthcare providers to focus on patient care.
- Medical assistants play a crucial role in improving patient care by managing administrative responsibilities.

Medical Reception:

- Medical receptionists set the tone for patient visits and handle various administrative tasks, including scheduling, registration, and communication.
- Efficient scheduling improves workflow and reduces patient wait times.

Patient Navigator/Advocate:

- As patient navigators/advocates, CMAs help patients navigate the healthcare system, coordinate care, and provide support beyond medical care.
- Effective communication is crucial in this role.

Medical Business Practices:

- Medical Business Practices bridge healthcare and administration, making the operation of healthcare facilities run smoothly.
- CMAs contribute to scheduling, organizing, medical records, billing, insurance processing, and compliance with healthcare regulations.

Establishing Patient Medical Records:

- Creating and maintaining patient medical records is essential for continuity and quality of care.
- CMAs must ensure patient data accuracy, confidentiality, and compliance with HIPAA regulations.

Scheduling Appointments and Practice Finances:

- CMAs manage appointment scheduling, balancing patient flow and provider time.
- They also play a role in practice finances, including financial reporting, insurance claims, and billing.
- Effective scheduling and financial management are interconnected, improving practice efficiency and financial health.

CHAPTER 3

Clinical Aspects

A Certified Medical Assistant's (CMA) job includes juggling patient care, administrative duties, and technical competence. A substantial chunk of this responsibility falls under clinical care, where CMAs play an important role in assisting healthcare practitioners and ensuring patients receive excellent treatment. This chapter will look at the different aspects of the CMA's clinical functions and responsibilities.

More Than Just Healthcare: Patient Interaction

Interaction with patients is the foundation of a CMA's clinical responsibilities. This engagement begins the moment a patient enters the hospital. As a CMA, you'll be the patient's initial point of contact, so you'll be in charge of providing a welcoming environment that can help them relax.

You will record patient histories, comprehend their concerns, and even explain procedures from here. To ensure that patients are informed, comfortable, and prepared for their visit, effective communication is vital throughout these exchanges.

Assisting with Exams and Procedures

CMAs frequently assist doctors and nurses during physical examinations and medical procedures. This can include everything from setting up the exam room and gathering the appropriate medical equipment to assisting the healthcare provider. CMAs may also conduct simple duties under the supervision of a healthcare physician in specific instances.

Collecting and Preparing Laboratory Specimens

Handling laboratory specimens is another important component of a CMA's clinical responsibility. CMAs may collect samples such as blood, urine, or tissues, according to state legislation and practice standards. After being collected, these samples are either tested in-house or readied for shipment to an outside laboratory. Understanding the proper methods for collection, storage, and transportation is critical for ensuring the accuracy of test results.

Conducting Basic Laboratory Tests

CMAs do basic laboratory testing in many healthcare settings. This includes routine urinalysis and running quick testing for illnesses such as strep throat or influenza. The accurate performance and interpretation of these tests are important for properly managing patients.

Administering Medications

Another critical clinical function of CMAs is to administer drugs as instructed by a healthcare physician. This necessitates a thorough awareness of the medications' purposes, doses, methods of administration, and potential side effects. Furthermore, CMAs must be aware of the legal and ethical implications of medicine administration.

Patient Education and Monitoring

Patient education is one of the important aspects when it comes to CMA's responsibilities. CMAs frequently advise patients on medication, food, lifestyle changes, and follow-up treatment. They may also phone patients to check on their progress and answer any issues they may have.

Infection Control and Safety Measures

Maintaining a safe environment is critical in the healthcare context. CMAs play a crucial role in executing infection control measures, which include appropriate hand hygiene, safe disposal of medical waste, sterilization of medical instruments, and following personal protective equipment rules.

The Scope of Clinical Practice

The clinical tasks of a CMA might vary substantially based on state legislation and the type of medical practice. Some CMAs specialize in a specific area of clinical practice, such as pediatrics or geriatrics, whereas others operate in a general practice and manage a variety of clinical activities.

To summarize, a CMA's clinical role is varied and dynamic. It is the heart of patient care, combining technical abilities, medical knowledge, and compassionate care. As a CMA, your clinical practice has a direct impact on patients rather than merely healthcare providers, making your involvement in healthcare delivery invaluable.

Patient Interview and Examination Room Techniques

In the fast-paced world of healthcare, Certified Medical Assistants (CMAs) frequently serve as the backbone, assisting the medical team in a variety of ways. Their responsibilities encompass several elements of patient care, including the Patient Interview and Examination Room Techniques. While these sectors have different needs, they all have the same end goal: to provide thorough, compassionate, and efficient patient care. In the following sections, we will look at the detailed processes, protocols, and communication skills required in both of these sectors to provide patients with the best healthcare experience possible.

Patient Interview: Building Bridges of Communication

A successful healthcare encounter is built on an excellent patient interview. It is the first point of contact for a Certified Medical Assistant (CMA), who gets vital information regarding the patient's current health concerns, medical history, lifestyle, and overall well-being.

Interviewing a patient necessitates a strong sense of empathy as well as outstanding communication skills. The goal is to provide a safe and open environment in which people can share their health issues and personal information. This is frequently accomplished through exhibiting respect for the patient's experiences, validating their feelings, and genuinely caring for their well-being. To begin, developing rapport is the foundation of a successful patient interview. This includes greeting the patient warmly, maintaining eye contact, and engaging in small talk to put them at ease. Remember that you set the tone for the patient's entire healthcare experience, so be courteous and nonjudgmental.

Following that, you must ascertain the patient's major complaint or the primary cause of their visit and ensure that what they say is written in their own words and accurately recorded in their medical record. After that, compile a complete history of the current illness (HPI). Ask open-ended questions to elicit a description of the patient's symptoms or problems, such as their onset, the frequency, the duration, and any things that affect them.

Next, investigate the patient's past medical history, which should include any chronic illnesses, hospitalizations, surgeries, and allergies. Also, remember to inquire about their family and social history, as well as lifestyle behaviors like smoking, alcohol consumption, food, and exercise, as these can have a significant impact on a person's health. The drug history is another important aspect when interviewing a patient.

Obtain a complete inventory of the patient's current medications, including prescription and over-the-counter medications and supplements they may be taking. To end the interview, summarize the information received and provide the patient the opportunity to clarify or add any additional information. This validates the data and allows individuals to feel heard and active in their care.

Examination Room Techniques: The Stage for Quality Healthcare

Following the completion of the patient interview, the following step in a CMA's clinical role comprises examination room techniques. This encompasses several activities, ranging from preparing the examination room to aiding during the examination.

Even before the patient reaches the examination room, the process begins. As a CMA, you must keep the room clean and organized and ensure supplies are equipped. This comprises examination gloves, gowns, drapes, and any specialized equipment required by the healthcare professional, such as a stethoscope, otoscope, or sphygmomanometer.

When the patient arrives, lead them into the examination room and give them specific instructions on what they must accomplish. If the patient is required to undress or wear a gown throughout the examination, make sure they understand the procedure while respecting their comfort and privacy.

During the examination, you may be required to hand instruments to the healthcare provider, hold and soothe the patient, or conduct responsibilities such as obtaining vital signs or reporting findings. Your specific responsibilities will vary depending on the demands of the healthcare professional, the type of examination, and the patient's condition.

The examination room technique includes sterilizing tools after procedures and properly disposing of medical waste. Avoiding the spread of infections ensures the safety of both patients and healthcare providers.

A CMA may also be required to clean and resupply the examination room after each patient. This comprises general cleaning activities, verifying that equipment is functioning properly, reporting any faults to the appropriate department, and maintaining a supply inventory.

Finally, good examination room strategies guarantee that medical treatments run easily and quickly. As a CMA, you are responsible for ensuring that the healthcare practitioner has everything they need and that the patient is comfortable and well taken care of during the examination. You make a substantial contribution to the quality of healthcare services delivered by implementing these practices.

Collecting and Processing Specimens

Medicine necessitates data, which frequently comes from within us in the form of diverse bodily specimens. The collecting and processing of these specimens is a crucial aspect of the work done by Certified Medical Assistants (CMAs), and it is required for diagnoses, treatment regimens, and overall patient health management.

Understanding the many specimens that can be collected, including but not limited to blood, urine, sputum, stool, and tissue samples, is the first step in mastering specimen-collecting techniques. Each instance can disclose a lot about a patient's health, but only if the model is effectively collected and analyzed.

Taking blood, for example, necessitates accuracy and expertise. Every step is critical, from verifying the patient's identity and explaining the procedure to applying the tourniquet, selecting the suitable needle, and puncturing the vein. The same holds true for urine collection, whether it is for a normal urinalysis or a clean-catch midstream specimen. Each process has characteristics that must be followed precisely to avoid cross-contamination or incorrect results.

Furthermore, specimen processing is just as important as obtaining them. It entails a number of duties, such as labeling, preparing for analysis, and storing or sending the models as needed.

Mislabeling can lead to serious mistakes in patient treatment, while incorrect preparation can jeopardize test results. It is the obligation of a CMA to scrupulously follow the guidelines and manage any unforeseen scenarios that may develop.

Blood samples, for example, must be centrifuged to separate serum or plasma from blood cells, whereas urine samples for a culture test must be frozen as soon as possible if not processed within an hour after collection. CMAs must be familiar with the onsite laboratory equipment and have a thorough understanding of the specimen processing guidelines.

Notably, safety is of the utmost importance throughout these operations. To safeguard themselves and their patients from potentially infectious materials, CMAs must follow Occupational Safety and Health Administration (OSHA) requirements. They must wear personal protective equipment, dispose of biohazard waste properly, and promote a clean environment.

Communication is also crucial. CMAs are frequently called upon to explain processes to patients, as well as address their worries and, in some cases, phobias. To calm a needle-phobic patient, for example, you could talk them through the procedure, use a smaller needle, or use a distraction tactic. As a result, the key to good specimen collecting and processing is a combination of technical abilities, safety precautions, and interpersonal interactions.

It's a measure of the healthcare industry's complexity that something as seemingly simple as collecting and processing specimens can include so many moving parts. Mastering these jobs, however, is part of CMAs' dedication to patient care because they represent the vital link between patients and the medical team. They typically go unnoticed since they labor behind the scenes, yet their contribution is critical in facilitating accurate diagnosis and effective treatments. Their attention to detail and dedication to their roles increase patients' trust in healthcare, transforming them into true unsung healthcare heroes.

Emergency Management/Basic First Aid

Emergency response and basic first aid are critical components of patient care in the healthcare system. When a life-threatening emergency happens, they are the first line of defense. These abilities are critical for Certified Medical Assistants (CMAs), as they frequently serve as the first responders before a patient visits a doctor or other healthcare practitioners.

Emergency Management: Making the Right Call

In an emergency, every second is important and can mean the difference between life and death. CMAs need to be trained to assess and respond to emergencies swiftly and appropriately. Emergency management starts with recognizing the situation. A patient's sudden chest pain, difficulty breathing, severe bleeding, or unconsciousness are clear signs of a medical emergency. CMAs must stay calm, promptly inform the physician, and ensure the emergency medical team is alerted if necessary.

Proper patient assessment plays a crucial role. Checking vital signs, keeping track of changes in the patient's condition, and documenting these observations accurately all feed into the medical team's intervention strategies. Moreover, CMAs should be equipped to use automated external defibrillators (AEDs) and administer cardiopulmonary resuscitation (CPR) if required. CMAs should be certified in BLS (basic life support) by the AHA (American Heart Association)

Basic First Aid: Immediate Care, Maximum Impact

Although it may appear easy, basic first aid can have a significant impact on a patient's well-being. The primary purpose is to stabilize the patient until more advanced medical therapy can be delivered. Simple measures, such as placing an unconscious patient in recovery to clear their airway, can have a big impact on their status.

Another critical part is understanding the fundamentals of wound care. Whether the wound is mild or serious, CMAs should know how to clean it, apply the appropriate dressing, and recognize the signs of infection.

Different degrees of burn necessitate different approaches. Cool water and a sterile dressing are usually enough to treat first-degree burns. More severe burns, on the other hand, necessitate rapid medical attention to manage pain and avoid infection. CMAs should be able to discriminate between burn severity and give appropriate first treatment.

Communication in Emergency Situations

In an emergency, communication is critical. CMAs must reassure and inform patients about their care while clearly and concisely communicating with other healthcare providers. This allows for improved decision-making and a smoother, more effective reaction.

Furthermore, in emergency situations, CMAs should comprehend the principles of the Incident Command System (ICS). This methodical approach to dealing with emergencies enhances response efficiency and ensures that every member of staff understands their job and duties.

Finally, CMAs must be familiar with emergency management and basic first aid. They are the initial line of defense in circumstances that require immediate action. CMAs play a vital role in improving patient outcomes and maintaining a high standard of care in their healthcare facilities by acquiring these skills.

Pharmacology

Pharmacology, the study of medications and their effects on the human body, is an important field of competence for a Certified Medical Assistant (CMA) as an integral component of the healthcare system. Understanding this topic is critical for pharmaceutical delivery that is safe and effective, patient education, and monitoring for potential side effects or adverse reactions.

Unraveling the Complex World of Drugs

There are numerous medications on the market, each with its own set of properties, modes of action, and potential interactions. CMAs should be knowledgeable about the key pharmacological classes, such as antibiotics, antihypertensives, antidiabetics, anticoagulants, and analgesics. CMAs can anticipate their effects, potential side effects, and any unique administration requirements by understanding these classes and their common representations.

Administration and Dosage

Medication administration is one of the key responsibilities of a CMA. In any healthcare context, the 'Five Rights' of pharmaceutical administration—the correct patient, drug, dose, route, and time—are non-negotiable. Even with simple drugs, mistakes in these areas can have major implications.

Dosages differ greatly amongst patients, based on age, weight, kidney function, and other medical issues. CMA will be able to avoid dosage errors and potential injury if they are aware of these issues and have a solid understanding of the medicine itself.

Drug Interactions and Contraindications

Drugs can interact with one another, with food, or with specific medical conditions, and these interactions can change how a drug works. Some interactions might either boost the desired therapeutic impact or cause undesirable side effects. Others can diminish the effectiveness of the medicine, potentially leading to treatment failure.

Knowing the common interactions of commonly used medications and recognizing when to raise concerns can help ensure patient safety. The same is true for contraindications, which are specific conditions or characteristics that render a specific drug or treatment inadvisable. With this information, CMAs can serve as an additional safety net in the healthcare team.

Patient Education and Advocacy

CMAs are frequently called upon to teach patients about their drugs. This task includes explaining what the drug does, why it is given, how it should be taken, and what adverse effects may occur in layman's words. This instruction is essential for ensuring patient adherence to their pharmaceutical regimen.

CMAs can also serve as patient advocates, observing and reporting harmful drug effects. CMAs can help ensure drugs serve their restorative goal without causing unnecessary harm by keeping a watchful eye and open lines of communication with patients.

Pharmacology is an important aspect of a CMA's training and daily duties. It is a complex, ever-changing field that necessitates continuous learning and close attention. CMAs play an important role in ensuring safe and effective pharmaceutical use in their healthcare settings, from drug knowledge and administration to patient education and advocacy. Their contributions in this domain have a direct impact on patient health outcomes, emphasizing the significance of their job and the need for their expertise.

Patient Education and Communication

Patient education and communication are critical factors in healthcare delivery. A Certified Medical Assistant (CMA) frequently serves as a key communication connection between healthcare professionals and patients, necessitating knowledge of educational principles as well as effective communication tactics.

Patient Education: Empowering through Knowledge

It is more than just explaining a diagnosis or treatment plan to a patient. It is about arming patients with the knowledge they need to make educated health decisions, understand their obligations, and actively participate in their care.

Medication instruction is one of the most important aspects of patient education. CMAs must explain to patients what each drug is for, how and when to take it, potential adverse effects to look out for, and any dietary or lifestyle changes that may be required.

Disease prevention and health promotion are also aspects of health education. Diet and nutrition, exercise, stress management, and preventive screenings are all topics that CMAs may cover. They may also teach patients with chronic conditions self-care skills, allowing them to better control their condition.

A successful patient education approach in all of these areas necessitates clear, succinct information provided in a manner that respects the patient's level of health literacy.

Mastering Communication

A vital thing to develop for successful patient education is communication. But what does this mean in a medical setting?

First and foremost, it necessitates active listening. When CMAs listen to a patient's concerns and questions, they demonstrate respect for the patient's experiences and establish a trustworthy relationship. Active listening also assists CMAs in understanding the patient's point of view, providing insight that can be used to direct educational efforts.

Second, successful communication entails communicating clearly and in a language that the patient understands. Medical jargon should be replaced with plain English. Visual aids, printed materials, and demonstrations can serve to supplement spoken explanations and assure comprehension.

Third, communicating entails evaluating for comprehension, which can sometimes be accomplished through the employment of the "teach-back" method, in which patients are asked to describe what they have been informed in their own words. This strategy enables CMAs to determine whether information has been understood and to clarify any misconceptions.

Finally, successful communication necessitates being attentive to a patient's feelings and demonstrating empathy. Because of this sensitivity, patients may feel more at ease asking questions and voicing concerns.

The Power of Non-Verbal Communication

Body language, tone of voice, and facial gestures can all transmit as much information as words. CMAs can reinforce their comments and contribute to a healthy communication environment by maintaining eye contact, assuming an open stance, and acting empathetically.

Navigating Cultural Differences

In an increasingly varied culture, CMAs may encounter patients from many ethnic origins. It is critical for effective communication and education to understand and accept cultural differences in health attitudes and practices. Cultural competency can help to avoid misunderstandings and promote a collaborative healthcare partnership.

Patient education and communication are at the heart of a CMA's function, whether explaining a prescription regimen, teaching a new self-care skill, or addressing a patient's concerns. CMAs who master these abilities can help to improve health outcomes, increase patient happiness, and contribute to a more efficient healthcare system. As the healthcare landscape evolves, the value of patient education and effective communication grows, emphasizing their critical role in a CMA's toolset.

Effective Communication

Effective communication in healthcare is more than a tool; it is a lifeline that connects all parties involved, develops healing connections, and facilitates optimal patient care. Certified Medical Assistants (CMAs) serve as the primary point of contact and are critical in keeping this lifeline operational.

The Cornerstones of Effective Communication

Clarity, respect, empathy, and active listening are the foundations of effective communication.

Clarity guarantees that the information presented is simple, exact, and medical jargon-free. It entails utilizing language that is appropriate for the patient's level of comprehension and health literacy.

Each interaction is founded on respect. Respecting the patient's rights, interests, preferences, and autonomy, as well as acknowledging that each patient actively participates in their healthcare journey, is essential.

Empathy, according to *Oxford*, is the ability to understand and share the feelings of another. Empathetic communication in a healthcare setting can help patients feel understood and supported, creating a therapeutic relationship.

Active listening entails fully concentrating on, comprehending, responding to, and remembering the words of a patient. It is critical for establishing trust, generating rapport, and comprehending the patient's point of view.

Verbal and Non-Verbal Communication

The use of words to convey information is known as verbal communication. In the context of healthcare, this can include describing a diagnosis, delivering prescription instructions, or discussing care plans.

Communication, however, entails more than just the spoken or written word. Nonverbal communication (e.g., body language, tone of voice, and facial expressions) is equally important. An open posture, for example, can express approachability, while sustained eye contact can demonstrate attentiveness, and a calm, soothing tone of speech can provide reassurance.

Effective Communication Across Different Mediums

Communication in the digital age expands beyond face-to-face contact. CMAs may be required to connect with patients via the phone, email, patient portals, or telemedicine platforms. Each medium has distinct characteristics that necessitate careful consideration. Telephone or telemedicine conversation, for example, lacks the visual clues that face-to-face contact provides, necessitating clear verbal communication and active listening.

Overcoming Communication Barriers

Healthcare communication can be hampered by a variety of factors, including linguistic or cultural difficulties, insufficient health literacy, fear or anxiety, and physical limitations such as hearing loss. To manage these hurdles, CMAs must be equipped with resources such as medical interpreters, educational materials, plain language, and assistive technologies.

Practice Your Communication Skills

Effective communication affects more than simply individual interactions; it also has an impact on broader areas of healthcare practice. For example, ensuring informed consent is critical, as patients want clear, full information to make educated decisions. It also plays a role in conflict resolution, where open, courteous discussion can aid in the resolution of differences and the maintenance of positive team dynamics.

The Impact of Effective Communication

Improved results in healthcare can be achieved through effective communication, which includes enhanced patient satisfaction, better adherence to treatment regimens, less patient anxiety, and improved health status. Furthermore, it has the potential to improve healthcare delivery efficiency and interprofessional collaboration.

To summarize, effective communication is a critical ability in any CMA's toolbox. It necessitates continual learning and practice, but it can result in significant gains in patient care and professional satisfaction. As healthcare becomes more patient-centered, the need for excellent communication will only increase, emphasizing the importance of acquiring this skill for any aspiring CMA.

Patient Education Principles

Patient education is critical in the healthcare system because it encourages the active participation of patients in their own care and making educated health decisions. It is critical for a Certified Medical Assistant (CMA) to comprehend and apply practical patient education techniques. This section will look at essential tactics and factors to consider when providing comprehensive patient education in a medical context.

Assessing Patient Needs

Before beginning any patient education, it is critical to examine the individual's needs, which include their medical condition, reading level, cultural background, and personal preferences. This assessment aids in tailoring the teaching approach to the patient's specific needs.

Clear Communication

Clear and succinct communication is essential for effective patient education. Avoid jargon and sophisticated medical terminology in favor of clear language that patients can grasp. To improve comprehension and promote discussion, use visual aids such as anatomical diagrams, charts, and models.

Health Literacy

According to the CDC, health literacy is "the degree to which individuals have the ability to find, understand, and use information and services to inform health-related decisions and actions for themselves and others." As a CMA, it is critical to assess patients' health literacy levels and adjust instructional materials. To ensure comprehension, simplify complicated concepts, give written materials at a suitable reading level, and encourage patients to ask questions.

Individualized Approach

Recognize that each patient is unique and that education must be tailored to each individual. Make teaching materials that are specific to the patient's ailment, treatment plan, and personal circumstances. Consider age, linguistic competence, cultural attitudes, and socioeconomic background while establishing instructional tactics.

Active Engagement

Engage patients in the learning process actively to improve their knowledge and retain information. Encourage patients to ask questions and provide them the chance to demonstrate their expertise through verbal or written explanations. To reinforce key concepts, use interactive teaching approaches such as role-playing or hands-on demonstrations.

Multimodal Teaching

To accommodate varied learning styles, use a variety of instructional approaches. Some patients prefer visual learning methods, while others prefer auditory or tactile methods. Use multimedia materials, such as movies or interactive web tools, to suit different learning styles and increase patient involvement.

Reinforcement and Follow-Up

Patient education should be a nonstop process, not a one-shot event. During following visits, reinforce essential facts and provide written resources for patients to refer to at home. Encourage patients to actively participate in their care by giving additional resources for further learning and assistance, such as trusted websites or support groups.

Cultural Sensitivity

When providing patient education, recognize and appreciate cultural differences. Be aware of cultural beliefs, customs, and health inequities that may influence a patient's comprehension and acceptance of medical knowledge. In order to achieve inclusivity and successful communication, incorporate culturally sensitive resources and adjust instructional approaches.

By following these patient education concepts, CMAs may establish a collaborative and empowering healthcare environment. Better health outcomes, higher patient satisfaction, and a stronger connection between patients and healthcare professionals are all benefits of effective patient education. As a CMA, your participation in patient education is critical to enhancing overall patient care and developing community health literacy.

Cultural Competence

Cultural competence is vital for Certified Medical Assistants (CMAs) in today's diversified healthcare environment. Understanding, respecting, and effectively communicating with people from various cultures is referred to as cultural competency. It entails identifying and treating patients' distinct beliefs, values, behaviors, and needs, resulting in a more inclusive and patient-centered approach to care. This section will discuss the significance of cultural competence in healthcare and techniques for CMAs to improve their cultural competence.

Relevance of Cultural Competence in Healthcare

Improved Communication and Trust

Cultural competency improves communication between healthcare workers and patients from various cultural backgrounds. Patients feel heard, appreciated, and understood when CMAs display cultural knowledge and respect. This results in trust development, which is essential for good healthcare delivery.

Enhanced Patient Engagement and Participation

Cultural competence empowers people to actively participate in their healthcare decisions. CMAs can include cultural beliefs, practices, and values in care plans when they take the time to learn about their patients' cultural views, practices, and values. By integrating patients into their care, CMAs enable patients to make educated decisions and take ownership of their health.

Reduction of Health Disparities

Cultural competence is critical in eliminating health disparities across various communities. CMAs can construct culturally relevant and responsive interventions by studying the cultural factors that influence health habits and access to care. This contributes to closing the healthcare outcomes gap across different cultural groups.

Strategies to Enhance Cultural Competence

Self-Reflection and Awareness

This is the first step in cultural competency development. CMAs should analyze their cultural biases, assumptions, and beliefs. This self-reflection increases self-awareness and sets the groundwork for recognizing and valuing cultural diversity in healthcare.

Cultural Humility

Recognizing that one's own cultural heritage may limit one's knowledge of others is an example of cultural humility. CMAs should approach conversations with humility, recognizing that they are constantly learning from patients and their different experiences. This approach encourages open-mindedness and adaptability to other cultural ideas.

Knowledge of Cultural Practices

CMAs should seek knowledge about the cultural practices and beliefs prevalent among their patients on a proactive basis. Understanding cultural norms on health, communication methods, dietary preferences, traditional therapeutic techniques, and religious or spiritual beliefs are all part of this. CMAs can provide culturally sensitive care if they are conversant with these factors.

Effective Communication

Cultural competence requires effective communication. CMAs should use simple language and avoid medical jargon or technical terminology that could confuse patients. It is also critical to be aware of nonverbal signs and body language, which might change among cultures and transmit various meanings.

Respect for Privacy and Modesty

Respecting cultural standards about privacy and modesty is essential for improving patient comfort and trust. CMAs should be aware of practices involving physical touch, eye contact, and gender-based care preferences. CMAs can provide a safe and courteous patient environment by tailoring their approach to local norms.

Collaboration and Teamwork

Individual contact with patients does not constitute cultural competency. CMAs should work with a diversified healthcare team that includes translators, cultural liaisons, and other experts who have knowledge of specific cultural norms. The healthcare team may guarantee that patient care is thorough and culturally responsive by working collaboratively.

Continuing Education

Cultural competency is a long-standing process. CMAs should actively seek chances for professional growth and instruction on cultural competency subjects. Attending workshops, participating in cultural competency training programs, or conducting self-study might help them gain a better knowledge of other cultures and healthcare disparities.

Feedback and Evaluation

CMAs should seek input from patients, colleagues, and supervisors to assess their cultural competence skills. These comments can assist in identifying areas for improvement and directing future professional growth. Regular self-evaluation and reflection are required to consistently improve cultural competency.

Finally, CMAs must be culturally competent in order to provide patient-centered treatment. CMAs may build trust, engagement, and improved health outcomes by embracing cultural diversity, practicing good communication, and respecting the views and values of patients from varied cultural origins. Cultural competency is a never-ending path that necessitates self-reflection, knowledge gain, and collaboration with various healthcare teams. By incorporating cultural competency into their practice, CMAs help to create a more inclusive and fair healthcare system.

Legal and Ethical Considerations

A Certified Medical Assistant's (CMA) duty involves key components of legal and ethical conduct within a healthcare setting, in addition to providing medical support. Understanding the intricacies of these concerns is critical for responsible and successful practice. This chapter delves into these crucial areas, providing a thorough examination of how CMAs must navigate the ever-changing landscape of medical ethics and law.

Understanding Legal Boundaries

The Importance of Scope of Practice

As a CMA, you must be aware of the legal boundaries that determine your scope of practice.' Each state defines this differently, dictating the tasks a CMA can undertake. Crossing these lines, whether consciously or unknowingly, may result in medical malpractice or negligence claims. Maintaining awareness of your stated function and tasks is thus a fundamental legal compliance component.

Confidentiality and Health Information Privacy

The Health Insurance Portability and Accountability Act (HIPAA) is important in the practice of a CMA. It requires the protection of patient privacy as well as the confidentiality of medical information. Violating any of these regulations may result in grave legal penalties. As a result, CMAs must be HIPAA compliant at all times, from secure data handling to maintaining patient confidentiality.

Ethical Considerations

Patient Autonomy and Informed Consent

Patient autonomy, or a patient's right to self-determination, is a sacred principle in healthcare. This value must be respected and upheld by CMAs. Informed consent is an important part of patient autonomy since it entails describing procedures, potential dangers, and benefits to patients and ensuring they have all the information they need to make decisions about their care.

Nonmaleficence and Beneficence

Nonmaleficence, which means "no harm," and beneficence, which requires medical practitioners to work in the best interests of the patient, are two more core ethical concepts in healthcare. These values remind CMAs of their responsibility to protect patients and prioritize their well-being.

Conflict Resolution

Legal and ethical considerations can sometimes appear to be at odds, resulting in moral quandaries. Knowing how to negotiate these situations is critical since they frequently necessitate a delicate balance of professional norms, personal morality, and legal obligations. In such cases, regular interaction with peers, mentors, and institutional ethical committees can provide invaluable insight.

Cultural Competence and Sensitivity

A CMA's job generally involves engaging with a wide range of patient demographics. As a result, demonstrating cultural knowledge and sensitivity is critical, as is honoring each patient's distinct cultural, societal, and personal values. Failure to do so may result in subpar care and legal and ethical breaches.

A CMA's job is filled with difficulties. It entails more than just competent medical aid; it necessitates a complete awareness of and adherence to legal and ethical standards. While norms and regulations may differ, ethical issues like as patient autonomy, nonmaleficence, and beneficence are universal. In order to offer quality patient care, a CMA must be proficient at navigating the medical landscape as well as the dense web of legal and ethical considerations.

Regulatory Guidelines for Certified Medical Assistants

In addition to the previously mentioned ethical and legal considerations, CMAs must follow regulatory rules established by federal, state, and professional authorities. These standards establish a solid framework for healthcare practices, directing CMAs to provide high-quality patient care while avoiding legal concerns.

Federal Regulations

HIPAA is the acronym for the Health Insurance Portability and Accountability Act.

HIPAA is a pillar of patient information protection. This federal regulation protects patients' privacy by limiting how medical information is stored, exchanged, and accessed. HIPAA's Privacy Rule, which protects individuals' medical records and other health information, and its Security Rule, which sets requirements for protecting health information maintained or transferred electronically, should be familiar to CMAs.

Occupational Safety and Health Administration (OSHA)

OSHA laws ensure workplace safety by enforcing infection control, hazard communication, and emergency preparedness standards. CMAs must follow these rules in order to offer an environment that is safe and healthy for patients and healthcare employees.

State Regulations

While federal restrictions apply throughout the country, state regulations might differ greatly. CMAs should comprehend the nuances of their state's practice rules, including but not limited to:

Medical Practice Acts

These state laws govern medical practice, including the scope of practice for medical assistants. They may decide what CMAs are and are not allowed to perform in their jobs, such as dispensing prescriptions, collecting vital signs, or assisting in small procedures.

State-specific Patient Privacy Laws

Some states may have privacy regulations that go beyond HIPAA's obligations, giving even stricter protection for specific types of health information. Adherence to these rules is crucial in order to avoid penalties and maintain patient privacy.

Professional Regulatory Guidelines

Regulatory rules and codes of behavior are also provided by professional organizations such as the American Association of Medical Assistants (AAMA). THE AAMA's Code of Ethics and Creed, FOR EXAMPLE, establishes values of honesty, respect, and professionalism, providing a road map for CMAs to navigate ethical and moral dilemmas.

Infection Control and Sterilization Guidelines

The Centers for Disease Control and Prevention (CDC) provides particular recommendations for infection prevention in healthcare settings in addition to OSHA's broad standards. These processes include hand hygiene, the use of personal protective equipment, the sterilization of medical instruments, and the disposal of medical waste.

The Importance of Continuing Education

Regulatory standards can and do change, necessitating CMAs' commitment to ongoing learning. As part of certification renewal, several states and professional organizations demand continuing education. These courses can keep CMAs up to date on the most recent legal, ethical, and professional standards, ensuring that their practice remains at the cutting edge of patient safety and care.

Navigating the complicated world of regulatory rules is essential to the function of a CMA. CMAs may assure the greatest standard of care and safeguard themselves, their patients, and their workplaces from potential legal and ethical infractions by being aware and compliant with these rules.

Medical Law and Ethics

Medical Law

Medical law is the foundation of healthcare practice, offering a solid framework of laws and regulations that healthcare practitioners, including Certified Medical Assistants (CMAs), must obey. The basic goal of medical legislation is to ensure that healthcare services are safe, efficient, and ethical.

Understanding Medical Malpractice

Medical malpractice is one of the most important parts of medical law. To prevent legal issues, CMAs must understand what constitutes malpractice, such as negligence. If a healthcare provider doesn't give a patient the level of care that a skilled and capable professional should provide in a similar situation and this leads to the patient getting hurt, it's considered a failure.

Informed Consent

Another important aspect of medical legislation is informed consent. A CMA must ensure that patients understand the procedure's aim, potential benefits and hazards, and alternative options before performing any medical procedure. Failure to get informed permission may result in legal consequences, such as charges of battery or negligence.

Mandatory Reporting

Certain scenarios, such as suspected child abuse, certain contagious diseases, or threats of self-harm, compel CMAs to disclose certain information. Failure to comply with mandated reporting regulations might result in legal implications and, in some situations, jeopardize patient safety.

Medical Ethics

While medical law establishes the legal framework for healthcare, medical ethics serves as the moral compass that guides CMAs' activities and judgments. In a healthcare setting, it entails making decisions about right or wrong, good or terrible.

Beneficence and Nonmaleficence

Beneficence, or the principle of doing good, encourages CMAs to take actions that help patients. Nonmaleficence, which is commonly characterized as "do not harm," compels CMAs to avoid causing harm to patients. These principles interact to remind CMAs of their fundamental commitment to enhancing patient health and well-being while reducing harm.

Autonomy and Respect for Persons

The notion of autonomy emphasizes the necessity of treating patients as persons capable of making informed health decisions. This notion is inextricably linked to informed consent, which is both a legal requirement and an ethical imperative to preserve patient autonomy.

Justice

In healthcare, the notion of justice refers to treating all patients equitably, regardless of age, ethnicity, gender, socioeconomic background, or disease state. CMAs must work hard to ensure that resources are distributed properly and that all patients have equitable access to healthcare and treatment options.

Confidentiality

Another ethical concept that is important in healthcare is confidentiality. Every patient has to keep their medical information private. CMAs must maintain this privilege by sharing patient information only when necessary and appropriate, such as for treatment or when required by law.

Finally, the interaction of medical law and ethics influences CMA roles and obligations. CMAs can negotiate the intricacies of healthcare by learning and following these principles, giving the greatest standard of care to their patients while preserving professionalism and legal compliance.

Summary

- Certified Medical Assistants have a multifaceted clinical role that involves patient care, administrative tasks, and technical skills.
- Patient interaction is a fundamental part of a CMA's clinical responsibilities, starting from welcoming patients and recording their histories to explaining procedures and ensuring their comfort.
- CMAs assist doctors and nurses during physical examinations and medical procedures, including preparing exam rooms and gathering medical equipment.
- They are responsible for collecting and preparing laboratory specimens, conducting basic laboratory tests, and administering medications following healthcare providers' instructions.
- Patient education, monitoring, and follow-up are essential aspects of a CMA's role, involving advising patients on medications, lifestyle changes, and treatment progress.
- Infection control and safety measures, such as hand hygiene and medical waste disposal, are crucial responsibilities to maintain a safe healthcare environment.
- The scope of a CMA's clinical practice can vary based on state regulations and medical practice type, with some specializing in specific areas like pediatrics or geriatrics.
- A CMA's clinical role combines technical skills, medical knowledge, and compassionate care, directly impacting patients' well-being and healthcare experience.
- Patient interviews are a critical part of a CMA's clinical duties, requiring empathy, communication skills, and the ability to build rapport.

- During patient interviews, CMAs gather essential information about the patient's health concerns, medical history, lifestyle, and well-being, aiming to create a safe and open environment for sharing.

- Key elements of a successful patient interview include developing rapport, documenting the patient's main complaint, obtaining a complete history of the current illness, and inquiring about past medical history, family and social history, lifestyle behaviors, and drug history.

- Summarizing the information and allowing patients to provide additional details or clarification at the end of the interview is essential for effective communication and patient-centered care.

- CMAs play a vital role in examination room techniques, from preparing the room with supplies to aiding during the examination.

- Keeping the examination room clean, organized, and well-equipped is crucial, including supplies like gloves, gowns, and specialized medical equipment.

- CMAs guide patients in the examination room, explain how the procedures work, and make sure that the patient is comfortable and their privacy protected.

- During examinations, CMAs assist healthcare providers, hand them instruments, obtain vital signs, and report findings.

- Sterilizing tools, disposing of medical waste, and cleaning and restocking the examination room are part of the examination room technique.

- Effective examination room techniques contribute to the quality and efficiency of healthcare services.

- Collecting and Processing Specimens:

- CMAs collect and process various bodily specimens, such as blood, urine, sputum, stool, and tissue samples.

- Accurate collection and analysis of specimens are essential for diagnoses, treatment plans, and patient health management.

- Proper techniques are required for collecting different types of specimens to avoid cross-contamination or incorrect results.

- Specimen processing, including labeling, preparation, and storage, is equally important for accurate testing.

- Safety measures, including compliance with Occupational Safety and Health Administration (OSHA) requirements, are crucial during specimen handling.

- CMAs must communicate effectively with patients about specimen collection procedures and address their concerns or phobias.
- CMAs serve as first responders in emergency situations, recognizing medical emergencies and initiating appropriate responses.
- They assess and document vital signs, provide CPR, and use automated external defibrillators (AEDs) when necessary.
- Basic first aid skills, including stabilizing patients and wound care, are crucial in emergencies.
- Effective communication and understanding of the Incident Command System (ICS) enhance emergency management.
- CMAs must be prepared to manage various emergencies and contribute to improved patient outcomes and care quality.
- CMAs require knowledge of pharmacology to ensure safe and effective medication administration.
- Understanding medication classes, dosages, administration routes, and potential interactions is essential.
- Medication administration follows the 'Five Rights' principle: correct patient, drug, dose, route, and time.
- CMAs play a role in patient education about medications, such as dosage, purpose, administration instructions, and side effects.
- Awareness of drug interactions, contraindications, and safety precautions is crucial.
- CMAs also monitor and advocate for patients regarding medication effects and potential adverse reactions.
- CMAs facilitate patient education by providing information, instructions, and resources.
- Patient needs, health literacy, and cultural background must be assessed before education begins.
- Effective communication includes clear, jargon-free language and the use of visual aids.
- Active engagement of patients through questions and interactive methods enhances learning.
- Multimodal teaching caters to different learning styles and preferences.
- Reinforcement, follow-up, and cultural sensitivity contribute to successful patient education.
- Effective communication involves respect, clarity, active listening, and empathy.
- Both verbal and non-verbal communication are vital in healthcare interactions.

- Communication across different mediums, such as phone or telemedicine, requires adapting to the medium's characteristics.
- Overcoming communication barriers, including language or cultural differences, is essential.
- Effective communication improves patient satisfaction, adherence to treatment, and healthcare delivery efficiency.
- Assessing patient needs, health literacy, and individual characteristics is essential.
- Clear communication in plain language and the use of visual aids promote understanding.
- Patient education should be individualized and engage patients actively.
- Multimodal teaching accommodates different learning styles.
- Continuous reinforcement, follow-up, and cultural sensitivity are key principles in patient education.
- Effective patient education empowers patients to make informed health decisions and enhances healthcare outcomes.
- Cultural competence improves communication, trust, patient engagement, and reduces health disparities in diverse healthcare settings.
- Self-reflection, cultural humility, knowledge of cultural practices, effective communication, respect for privacy, collaboration, continuing education, and feedback are essential for cultural competence.
- CMAs must understand legal boundaries, ensure confidentiality, uphold ethical principles, and show cultural sensitivity in their healthcare practice.
- CMAs should comply with federal, state, and professional regulations, including HIPAA, OSHA, state-specific laws, professional codes of ethics, infection control, and sterilization guidelines. Continuing education is vital.
- CMAs must steer clear of making medical mistakes, make sure patients understand and agree to treatments, report when necessary, and follow ethical guidelines such as doing good for patients, avoiding harm, respecting patient choices, treating everyone fairly, and keeping medical information private.

CHAPTER 4
Anatomy And Physiology

CMAS ARE NOT required to function as doctors or even to execute the responsibilities that doctors do. They are, nevertheless, expected to have a rudimentary knowledge of the human body as well as some medical facts. This section will cover the subjects of human anatomy and physiology. Human anatomy is essentially the study of a person's structure and formation. It entails an awareness of the fundamental body parts that allow humans to function. At the same time, we will look at human physiology, which is basically the physics behind how the human body works and functions.

Understanding the illness process requires an understanding of anatomy. Anatomy, in addition to explaining anatomical components, teaches about surgical planes for dissection, muscle motions, joint function, and damage processes. With imaging tests being used routinely to diagnose disorders, healthcare workers must grasp cross-sectional anatomy and how it relates to function and disease. The following body systems are important to understand:

Cardiovascular System

The heart is the most important part of our body. It is placed slightly on the left side of your chest and is protected from external injury by the chest wall and ribs. It's responsible for pumping and circulating blood throughout the body. The heart ensures that blood is given to all regions of the body by contracting and expanding muscles.

The heart is entirely formed of muscles and is around the size of your fist. The heart has three layers that protect its activities while also ensuring its strength to sustain continuous contractions. The epicardium is the outer layer, which is followed by the myocardium and endocardium on the inside.

The interior cavity of the heart is separated into four chambers. These are the right and left atriums and the right and left ventricles. The atria are the thin-walled chambers, while the ventricles are the thick-walled chambers. The superior and inferior vena cava are like the drains that deoxygenate blood from the body and bring it back to the right atrium. Deoxygenated blood then enters the right atrium, then into the right ventricle, and is carried to the lungs through the pulmonary artery.

Following oxygenation, blood is returned to the left atrium via the pulmonary veins. It subsequently enters the left ventricle and is pumped to the remainder of the body via the aorta.

- There are four valves in the heart—tricuspid, mitral, aortic, and pulmonary. These valves keep blood from flowing backward.
- The septum separates the heart chambers in the middle.
- The aorta is the largest vessel for blood in the body, and it delivers oxygenated blood.
- The pericardium is a protective fibrous layer that wraps around the heart.
- Arteries carry oxygenated blood out from the heart and to tissues (arteries away).
- Veins transport deoxygenated blood from the tissues back to the heart.
- Erythrocytes are red blood cells that carry oxygen.
- Leukocytes are white blood and fight infection.
- Systole is the activation or pumping of the heart.
- Diastole is when the heart relaxes.
- A murmur is an irregular sound heard in the heart.
- Carotid arteries can be palpated in the neck. They supply blood to the brain.
- The SA node, located in the right atrium, is the heart's pacemaker.

Central Nervous System

The human brain is a complex and intricate organ that has developed to control nearly every function in the body. Over 1,000 billion nerves in the human brain are used for a variety of bodily processes. To support human physiological activities, these nerves deliver messages to all parts and regions of the body.

Aside from terminating impulses to all regions of the body, the brain also performs the critical functions of emotions and memory. Given the brain's critical role in coordinating bodily functions, it is an essential organ that must be protected. CMAs, like all other medical practitioners, must learn how to protect the body.

Many different tissues and fluids compose the brain. The cerebrum makes up most of the brain's structure. Its tissue generates chambers that contain a fluid known as cerebrospinal fluid. The brain is divided into three sections: the forebrain, the midbrain, and the hindbrain. Although they all have the same appearance, they perform various functions.

Here are the primary regions of the brain and their functions:

- Cortex: The cortex is the brain's outer layer, like its surface. It serves as the beginning point for brain activities like movement.
- The Brainstem: This is the section of the brain at the bottom. It regulates vital functions like sleep, blood pressure, and breathing.
- The Cerebellum: This region of the brain is located at the bottom. The cerebellum regulates functions such as body balance, gait, and mobility.
- The Basal Ganglia: This is the brain's command center, responsible for delivering messages and signals to different regions of the body. The basal ganglia are located in the core of the brain.

The brain is further subdivided into lobes, each with its special and distinct functions. The following are the brain's primary lobes:

1. Frontal Lobe: The frontal lobes are responsible for a person's problem-solving abilities. The frontal lobes also regulate a person's motor function, cognitive function, and emotions.
2. Occipital Lobe: The occipital lobe is involved in vision and aids in the conversion of visual impulses from the eye into an image.
3. Temporal Lobes: The temporal lobes are in charge of a person's hearing, scent, and memory.
4. Parietal Lobes: The parietal lobe controls a person's senses, including speech. It controls and adjusts sensory activities all over the body.

Other aspects of the Central Nervous System:

1. The pituitary gland is in charge of producing various hormones, including vasopressin, oxytocin, and thyroid and adrenal hormone-stimulating factors.
2. The sympathetic and parasympathetic nervous systems are the two divisions of the autonomic system. The autonomic nervous system is responsible for involuntary functions like digestion, heartbeat, and breathing. The sympathetic is generally responsible for "fight

or flight" responses and the parasympathetic is generally responsible for "rest and digest" functions.

3. There are 12 cranial nerves that control face movements, speech, swallowing, vision, and other functions.

4. There are 33 vertebrae in the spinal cord. The vertebrae come together to form the vertebral column, which protects the spinal cord and major nerves. Nerves escape through microscopic holes in the vertebrae to supply the body components.

5. The cerebrospinal fluid envelops the brain, shielding it from whatever harm.

6. The Glasgow Coma Scale is used to assess the level of consciousness. It includes 3 aspects: eye-opening, verbal response, and motor response.

7. An EEG, which measures brain waves, is done in individuals who are suspected of having seizures.

8. The hypothalamus regulates sleep, appetite, and temperature.

9. A lumbar puncture is a procedure that collects CSF samples to test for infection (specifically meningitis), malignancy, or hemorrhage.

Endocrine System

The endocrine organs produce hormones that are essential for growth, development, and electrolyte and blood glucose balance. Even though the endocrine glands are located outside the brain, several of these glands are controlled by pituitary and hypothalamic hormones.

1. ACTH is produced by the pituitary gland. It stimulates the adrenal gland to produce corticosteroids.

2. The anterior (front part) pituitary gland releases LH and FSH. They enhance spermatogenesis and oogenesis by acting on the ovaries and testes. The male sex hormone testosterone is required for sexual trait development.

3. Gluconeogenesis is the process through which glucose is produced in the liver. Glycogen is a substance formed from glucose and stored in the liver.

4. The anterior pituitary gland secretes growth hormone, which is needed to achieve growth and development. Acromegaly can be caused by excessive GH secretion.

5. Prolactin, another hormone released by the anterior pituitary, helps in the production of milk in the breast.

6. The posterior pituitary gland releases vasopressin or ADH. It helps with fluid equilibrium and urine production. Diabetes insipidus is characterized by the absence of ADH. This causes an increase in urine production.

7. The pineal gland is a small neuronal organ in the brain. Melatonin, which regulates the sleep-wake cycle, is known to be secreted.

8. Parathyroid hormones play a role in calcium regulation.

9. The thymus is located directly behind the upper sternum. This gland aids in the generation of T lymphocytes.

10. Epinephrine is released by the adrenal medulla, and corticosteroids are secreted by the adrenal cortex. Addison's disease can be caused by a lack of or insufficient adrenal gland activity. Cushing syndrome is caused by excessive corticosteroid secretion.

11. The pancreas helps in the production of insulin and glucagon. Insulin makes blood sugar levels lower, whereas glucagon boosts them. Polydipsia means having an extreme or excessive thirst, while polyphagia refers to an excessive or heightened appetite. Diabetes mellitus is caused by a lack of or resistance to insulin. Type 1 diabetes occurs when the patient's body cannot produce insulin. Type 2 diabetes develops when the patient can produce insulin but is resistant to it. A1c is an abbreviation for glycosylated hemoglobin, used today for diabetes monitoring and diagnosis.

Gastrointestinal System

1. It begins with mechanical and chemical food breakdown so that little food particles can be absorbed.

2. Food is eaten in the mouth, followed by chemical digestion. Amylase, an enzyme that breaks down carbs, is found in saliva.

3. Food is subsequently forced down the esophagus. At the same moment, the epiglottis folds over and wraps the larynx to block food from entering the airways. The muscles of the esophagus drive food down into the stomach.

4. The food is mixed with gastric acids in the stomach, and the protein is digested. The discharge of hydrochloric acid from the stomach cells lining its wall aids digestion.

5. The partially digested and broken food next enters the small intestine, which consists of the jejunum, duodenum, and ileus. Many enzymes in the small intestine can digest fat, protein, and carbs. The small intestine is where the majority of the meal is absorbed.

6. Foods that are absorbed in the small intestine now transfer into the large intestine via the ascending or right colon. At this point, the food has the consistency of feces. It then enters the transverse colon, followed by the descending colon. Water is absorbed by the colon, including electrolytes.

7. The fecal matter then enters the rectum. When there is a defecation reflex, the anal sphincters relax, and the anus empties.

The liver is another vital human organ. The human liver performs numerous tasks, and any issue that interferes with these functions might be fatal. The liver can be located in the upper right quadrant of the abdomen and is shielded from external harm by the ribs. It is one of the largest organs in the body and has numerous tasks. The liver's primary function is to synthesize and digest nutrients.

The liver has the right and left lobes, each having its own set of functions. Although both lobes execute filtration functions, they do so on separate terms. The liver serves as a detoxification center in addition to being a filter. It aids the body's metabolization of medications and substances that may otherwise be harmful.

The liver secretes bile while executing its function, which ends up in the stomach. Bile is stored in the gallbladder and is necessary for fat digestion and emulsification.

Respiratory System

A group of organs that help with breathing by exchanging oxygen and excreting carbon dioxide. The lungs are found on both sides of the chest known also as the thorax. The lungs are spongy and filled with air. The trachea, often known as the windpipe, transfers the air we use for breathing to our lungs. The bronchi are a tubular network that transports air. Bronchioles are significantly tiny units that separate the tubes for the passage of oxygen.

Bronchioles carry air into microscopic air sacs called alveoli, which are bordered by capillaries. In the alveoli, these arteries take oxygen while releasing carbon dioxide. Exhaled is the carbon dioxide that has been expelled into the air sacs. In humans, the regular process of breathing is created by inhaling and exhaling air. The Respiratory Center can be found in the Pons.

The lungs' primary function is to deliver oxygen to the blood. They also release carbon dioxide. When the lungs are working properly, a person should have no trouble breathing. A number of issues may arise if the lungs have issues. This usually signifies that the rest of the body will receive insufficient oxygen.

The lungs are divided into lobes, with tissue separating each lobe from the next. While the left lung is divided into two, the right lung is divided into three lobes.

The respiratory system's parts

- Mouth and nose
- Sinuses
- Pharynx
- The trachea links the back of the neck to the lungs (sometimes referred to as the "windpipe") and plays a vital role in the respiratory system by allowing air to flow between the larynx and bronchi.
- Bronchus
- Lungs
- Alveoli—where gas exchange occurs
- The pleura is the membrane surrounding the lungs

The nose, pharynx, and larynx are all part of the upper respiratory system.

The trachea, bronchial tree, and lungs comprise the lower respiratory system.

The contraction of muscles such as the diaphragm allows air to enter the lungs.

The respiratory system also performs the following functions, aside from gas exchange:

- Allows you to talk
- Warms and moisturizes the inhaled air
- Delivers oxygen to the tissues
- Protects the airways from foreign substances

Many conditions affect your respiratory system, namely as follows:

- Allergic reactions
- Atelectasis is a lung collapse.
- Allergies
- Infections such as pneumonia
- Diseases such as COPD, emphysema, and bronchitis
- Cancer
- Effusions: the gathering of fluid in the chest cavity
- Pneumothorax: an air accumulation in the chest cavity
- Pulmonary edema: a condition in which fluid builds up inside the lung tissues
- Pulmonary embolism: a condition where a blood clot blocks the pulmonary artery

Tuberculosis is an illness of the lungs caused by the bacteria Mycobacterium tuberculosis.

Skeletal System

There are two sections in the skeletal system: the appendicular system and the axial system.

The axial system consists of the following:

- Skull bones, which include facial bones
- Bones located in the middle ear
- The rib cage
- Vertebrae and sternum

The appendicular system consists of the following:

- Arm and forearm bones such as the ulna, radius, and humerus
- Scapula and clavicle
- The hand, as well as all of the finger bones
- Pelvis (including hips)
- The thigh and legs, which include the fibula, femur, patella, and tibia.

o   Ankles and feet

1. The skeletal system's primary responsibilities are to protect, support, and aid in body mobility. It also helps to produce red blood cells in the bone marrow (center of the bone).

2. Cartilage is found in all joints; it is made up of dense connective tissue and serves to protect the joints from harm.

3. Tendons connect muscle to bone, while ligaments connect bone to bone.

4. Ossification is the process through which bone is formed.

5. Osteomalacia refers to bone softening.

6. Calcium and vitamin D both influence bone development.

7. Smoking and drinking both inhibit calcium absorption.

8. Osteoporosis is the weakening of bone, which makes it brittle. Listed are common risk factors for osteoporosis:
   o   Female sex
   o   Fair skin
   o   Postmenopausal

9. Osteoarthritis occurs when there is cartilage loss and chronic inflammation of the bones within a joint.

10. Gout occurs when there is uric acid accumulation in the joint.

11. A humpback is characterized by kyphosis, while a lateral curvature of the spine is characterized by scoliosis.

Urinary System

Kidneys are paired organs that look like beans. They are located on either side of the midline abdomen and serve an important function in waste removal. The kidneys ensure that the blood and other body fluids are properly balanced through the filtration process. What is in urine is 95% water, and the rest is trash (5%).

Each kidney has approximately 1,000 microscopic filters called nephrons. As long as the kidney is healthy, the nephrons stay active throughout a person's life. However, there is a chance that the nephrons will be injured. If the nephron is deprived of blood for several hours, the kidney can perish. The kidney cannot regenerate after it has died. To help the patient live normally again, the only choice is to conduct a kidney transplant.

The kidneys, bladder, urethra, and ureters comprise the urinary system. While performing its waste clearance function, the system also regulates blood pressure. Furthermore, the urinary system aids in the creation of erythropoietin, a chemical that aids in the formation of bone marrow. The urinary system organs also serve acid-balancing and fluid-conservation responsibilities. The urinary system's primary organs and their functions are listed below.

Kidneys: The kidney is the primary and most essential organ of the urinary system. Every human has two kidneys. Because of the existence of the liver, the right kidney is normally placed a few centimeters lower than the left kidney. The adrenal gland secretes the hormone aldosterone, which regulates salt reabsorption from the renal tubules. The pituitary hormone ADH regulates water excretion by the kidneys. Renin is an enzyme that the kidneys make. This regulates blood pressure.

Ureters: The ureters are the second organs that comprise the urinary system. The ureters are two tubes in the body. They are responsible for the transportation of urine from the kidneys to the bladder. The ureters move urine into the bladder by squeezing their muscles.

The bladder is a tiny triangular-shaped organ located in the lower abdomen. The bladder is in charge of retaining urine. The bladder walls are extremely elastic and can stretch to accommodate enormous volumes of urine. When a person urinates, the walls of the bladder expand and compress to push the pee out. A healthy adult's bladder should be able to store up to two cups of urine for up to five hours.

Nerves: Nerves are essential for kidney function. Nerves in the urinary system control the function of the bladder and urethra. The nerves warn a person of the need to urinate and also aid in the control of urine flow.

The Urethra: In the center of the urethra is a short tube-like structure that joins the urinary meatus and the bladder. When one empties the bladder, the urethra serves as a valve and opens. It is controlled by the nerves.

Sphincter Muscles: These are the muscles that prevent pee from spilling from the bladder accidentally. Because the bladder lacks valves, urine would easily leak out if the muscles at its opening were lax. The sphincter muscles seal over the bladder entrance, allowing urine to flow outside the urethra to be controlled.

Reproductive System

The reproductive system not only produces sex hormones, but it is also in charge of the generation of sperm cells and eggs. It is also in charge of transporting the fertilized egg through the fallopian tube to the uterus for implantation. The reproductive system is also involved in hormone production and the development of the fetus. Different organs in the body perform these fundamental reproductive system processes. It is vital to highlight that the reproductive organs in men and women have different functions.

The Female Reproductive System

There are much more in the female reproductive system than in the male. To begin, the female reproductive system is in charge of the generation of egg cells. The system is also responsible for delivering the eggs via the fallopian tube to the moment of fertilization. The sperm normally comes into contact with the eggs in the fallopian tube, where the initial fertilization occurs. The female reproductive system has two parts: internal and exterior.

The Internal Female Reproductive System

The internal female reproductive system consists of three important organs: the vagina, ovaries, and uterus. The ovaries contribute to egg cell production, and the uterus houses the fertilized egg.

The Vagina

The vagina is a hollow and muscular tube that runs from the pubic area to the uterus's end. The muscular walls flex and extend as needed to keep the vagina moist and allow it to perform its functions. Among the important tasks played by the vagina are as follows:

o   Allows the penis to penetrate during sexual intercourse.

o   aids the child's transition from the uterus to the outside world during birth.

o   Aids with the passage of blood during menstruation.

o   The vagina is protected by a thin lining called the hymen. This lining is preserved until a lady has her first sexual contact.

The Uterus

The uterus protects the fertilized egg up until it becomes a baby. The uterine walls are very elastic, allowing it to expand and shrink. It allows a kid to grow inside the womb and promotes the child's well-being. During labor, the uterine walls assist in pushing the baby out.

The Fallopian Tubes

The fallopian tubes are hollow, thin structures that link the ovaries to the uterus. They protrude from the top of the uterus. The fallopian tubes are responsible for transferring the ovum from the ovaries to the place of fertilization. The ovum is delivered to the uterus after fertilization, where it will implant and mature.

The Ovaries

The ovaries are oval-shaped organs that are located on both ends of the uterus. The ovaries play critical roles in egg production and storage. When an egg is created, the ovaries carry it down the fallopian tubes to where it is fertilized.

External Female Reproductive Organs

In addition to internal reproductive organs, the female reproductive system has exterior organs. These are the organs:

Labia Minora: The tiny labia are two-inch-long organs found inside the labia majora. The urethra, which is a tube that transports urine from the bladder on its way out, surrounds the organs.

Labia Majora: The fleshy coating that shields the internal organs from damage is referred to as the labia majora. The labia majora includes sweat and oil glands. These glands are in charge of keeping the reproductive system lubricated.

Clitoris: The clitoris is the point at which the two labia minoras meet. It protrudes similarly to the penis, with the labia minora serving as its scrotum. The clitoris is a highly sensitive organ that influences sexual excitement.

The Male Reproductive System

Male reproductive systems differ from female reproductive systems. Males, unlike females, do not have a uterus, fallopian tubes, or ovaries. The penis, testicles, duct system, and glands compose the male reproductive system.

Accessory Glands: The male reproductive system includes a number of accessory glands. These are the vesicles and the prostate glands. The glands create a variety of fluids required by the male reproductive system. These glands' secretions are also necessary for feeding sperm.

The Duct System: The duct system is in charge of sperm movement. The vas deferens and the epididymis comprise this system.

Testicles: In males, the testicles are oval-shaped structures that produce millions of sperm. They are critical in ensuring that the male reproductive system performs optimally.

The penis. The penis is an external male reproductive organ composed of highly specialized expanding and contracting muscles. The primary components of the penis are the shaft and the glans. The glans are the penis's head, and the shaft is the tubular section. The major function of the penis in reproduction is to transport the sperm cell to the egg cell. The penis penetrates the vagina during sexual contact. Sperm cells are discharged during the procedure and fertilize the ovum.

Roles Played by the Male Reproductive System

The male reproductive system is not as active as the female reproductive system, yet it is important in reproduction. Among the reproductive system's functions to be noted are sperm cell formation, sperm production, and the production of male sex hormones, which indicate whether a man is mature enough to participate in sexual activity.

Every day, an adult guy creates millions of sperm cells. The seminiferous tubules are crucial in the production of sperm cells. When a man reaches puberty, the sex hormones he produces convert the cells in his seminiferous tubules into sperm cells. The sperm cell develops into a tadpole with a tail. This sperm cell is responsible for fertilizing the egg produced by the ovaries.

Sperm Cell Storage and Transmission

When a sperm cell matures, it is moved to the vas deferens, also known as the sperm duct. The sperms combine with the fluids produced by the different glands, particularly the vesicle glands, in the sperm duct. The seminal fluid is the major fluid created by the seminal vesicles and is usually stimulated during sexual contact. The stimulation causes the penis to stiffen in preparation for sexual intercourse.

The stimulation of the sperm continues during sexual intercourse. The muscles of the male reproductive system eventually contract, forcing out the sperm. This is referred to as ejaculation. Millions of sperm are expelled when a male ejaculates into a female vagina. These sperms compete for the ovum, which is normally still within the fallopian tubes. The first sperm to reach the ovum fertilizes it and prevents the other sperm cells from entering.

Hormonal Influence

1. The sex hormones LH, FSH, and testosterone are required by both the male and female reproductive systems.
2. The Synthesis of sperm requires FSH.
3. LH promotes the synthesis of testosterone

4. For male sexual characteristics to grow, such as strength, sex drive, and bone mass, testosterone is required.

5. Progesterone and estrogen are female sex hormones.

Integumentary System (Nails, Hair, Skin, and Glands)

1. The epidermis is the skin's outermost and most superficial layer.

2. The dermis is the layer of skin just beneath the epidermis that contains glands, blood vessels, and hair follicles.

3. A Macule is a flat lesion that is less than 0.5 cm in diameter.

4. A Patch is a flat lesion that is greater than 0.5 cm in diameter.

5. A papule is a raised lesion that is less than 0.5 cm in diameter.

6. A nodule is a raised lesion that is larger than 0.5 cm in diameter.

7. A cyst is a semi-solid lesion that is spherical.

8. A plaque is a solid raised lesion that is larger than 0.5 cm in diameter.

Common Skin Disorders

1. Contact dermatitis: a condition characterized by itching and dry skin after contact with an irritant.

2. Xerosis: dry skin commonly found in the elderly.

3. Hemangioma: a vascular birthmark characterized by visible blood vessels.

4. Melanoma: A deadly skin cancer that is exacerbated by sunshine.

5. Shingles, or herpes zoster, is a childhood ailment.

6. Cold sores around the lips and genitals are caused by Herpes simplex.

7. Scratching causes excoriations on the skin.

Surgical and Medical Patient Positions

Several positions are used to assess patients during medical exams and surgeries. The position chosen is determined by the surgery and the surgeon's preferences. Other aspects to consider during the surgical placement of the patient include the length of the procedure, the kind of anesthetic, and access to the arms/legs for IV medicine administration. A safety belt or strap is always utilized to secure the patient, regardless of position. Before placing a patient in any surgical position, the following should be known:

- Patient Age
- Mobility
- Skin Condition
- Weight
- Joint Limitation
- Pre-existing Medical Conditions
- Patient Privacy

There are various patient postures, each with minor variations:

- Supine (face up)
- Prone (face down)
- Trendelenberg (supine with bed angling the head lower than the feet)
- Lateral Decubitus (side lying)
- Lithotomy (supine with legs bent and open—for OB-GYN/pelvic exams)
- Jackknife (prone, bent at the waist)
- Sims (side lying with arm and leg extended)
- Semi fowler (bed angled so the patient is sitting up with legs extended)

Supine

- The patient is lying on his back, face, and abdomen pointing to the ceiling, arms at his sides or abducted (moved away from the body) to 90 degrees, palms facing up.
- A pillow is frequently inserted behind the knees and padding is placed under the head, arms, and heels.
- The supine position is commonly used for surgery on the chest, abdomen, and face area, and it has resulted in a decrease in mortality owing to Sudden Infant Death Syndrome.

Prone

- In this position, the individual lies on his or her stomach, with the back to the ceiling. This is a frequent posture during neck or back surgery. Because the face can be crushed against the mattress or bed frame, it is usually protected.
- Ensure that the genitals are not crushed during surgery on patients in the prone position. As a result, a pillow or a roll is frequently tucked directly beneath the pubis.

Lithotomy

- This position has multiple variants Image depicting the conventional lithotomy position
- It is frequently used to inspect the pelvis and lower abdomen.
- The patient is to be laid in a supine position on the table, hips extended and knees flexed.
- Special tools (stirrups) are used to hold the legs up. This type of position is commonly employed by urologists to access the genitals and bladder, and by gynecologists to access the perineum.
- This posture is also used by general surgeons to gain access to the lower colon and rectum.
- Prolonged placing of patients in the lithotomy position, on the other hand, may result in nerve injury or vascular compromise (compartment syndrome).
- Before placing the patient in the lithotomy position, he or she should be unconscious. When placed in the lithotomy position, patients experience a loss of control and an increased sensation of vulnerability.

Semi fowler

- In the Semi-Fowler's position, the patient rests flat on the bed with the back elevated and the legs straight or bent.

Fowler position

- In Fowler's position, the patient sits or lies on the bed with the head and upper body elevated at various angles, often 45 to 60 degrees.

- Fowler's position is often employed in post-operative patients, stroke patients in danger of aspiration, and heart failure patients because it allows the patient to cough and makes breathing easier. It is also a beneficial position for patients in respiratory distress since it allows for easier breathing.
- Fowler's posture is frequently used in postpartum females to allow for perineum drainage.
- This posture is frequently used in patients who are fed through oral or nasogastric tubes because it lowers the risk of aspiration. Gravity influences both swallowing and peristaltic action.

Trendelenburg position

- The patient is positioned supine (on their back). Their heads were down, and their feet were elevated above the level of their head.
- A bed or table tilt of 10–25 degrees with the head lowered is typical.
- To facilitate surgical site access, it is commonly utilized in surgery, particularly in abdominal and pelvic procedures.
- The tilt forces abdominal organs upward, improving surgical visibility.
- Secure patients to minimize slippage, utilize proper padding, and provide safety and comfort support.
- It has the potential to disrupt venous blood return, which could have medical consequences.
- Because of diaphragm displacement, the position can affect respiratory function.
- Patients in the Trendelenburg posture must be closely monitored.

Jackknife Position (also referred to as the Kraske position)

- The patient is positioned on the abdomen, and the bed is flexed at the hips. This causes the head to drop and the buttocks to rise.
- This allows easy access to the anal region, buttocks, and lower back. It is frequently prescribed to treat hemorrhoids, anal fissures, and pilonidal illnesses.
- The technique can also be utilized to gain access to the sacrum, buttocks, and perianal regions.
- Typically, the patient is put to sleep first, then turned over in the jack knife position. To confirm that there is no compression, the eyes, face, and genitals must be examined.

Sim's Position

- This position, also known as the left lateral position, is frequently used to inspect the rectum, administer enemas, and assess women with vaginal prolapse.
- The patient is lying on his left lateral side.
- Straighten the left hip and lower leg and flex the right hip and knee.
- There is excellent access to the rectum and anal region.
- It is a highly safe and comfortable position for the patient.

Caution

The following general precautions should be taken regardless of the type of patient position chosen:

- Always assess the patient's overall health prior to positioning
- Keep in mind that a patent airway is required
- Avoid excessive pressure from bones on the hard surface
- Ensure the body's circulation and perfusion are intact
- Check to ensure that the position provides adequate exposure to the relevant body part
- Ensure the patient is comfortable and safe
- Avoid nerve stretching and compression
- Record the patient's neurovascular status before, during, and after the procedure

Common Anatomical Terms to Describe the Location

Certain words must be understood while addressing the patient's anatomy and axis/plane. Among them are the following:

Anterior: Refers to the patient's front (a.k.a. ventral)

Posterior: Refers to the patient's back; it is also known as dorsal

Superior: Towards or on top of the head. It is also known as cranium.

Inferior: Refers to the lower body (a.k.a. caudal)

Medial: refers to the direction of the body's center or middle.

Lateral: Located away from the body's midline or to the flanks.

Proximal: Means close. The mouth, for example, is considered proximate.

Distal: Means far away: The anus, for example, is considered distant.

Volar: A word that is frequently used to describe the underside of the foot (the sole) or the palm of the hand.

Dorsum: Means to the back of the hand.

Contralateral: Means the opposite side. A patient, for example, may have swollen lymph nodes on the opposite side.

Ipsilateral: Refers to being on a similar side. A patient, for example, may have a lesion on the neck as well as swollen axillary lymph nodes on the same side.

Deep: Situated further away from the surface. An individual, for example, may have a large collection of pus.

Superficial: Refers to being close to the surface. For instance, the patient could have sustained a minor wound to the hand caused by a knife. The damage caused by superficial wounds is usually minor.

Anatomical Planes

Planes are frequently used to explain anatomy. This refers to two-dimensional bodily sections. Because CT scans and other imaging modalities produce images in planes, it is critical to understand the terminology.

The sagittal plane

1. Vertically parts the body into left and right sides.
2. A median plane is a vertical plane in the middle.
3. The parasagittal plane is formed when the sagittal plane divides the body into uneven portions.

The frontal plane divides the body into two segments: anterior (front) and posterior (back).

The *transverse plane* separates the body horizontally into upper and lower halves. CT scans often examine the body in transverse planes.

Anatomical Terms to Describe Muscles and Their Attachments

The majority of muscle arises from bone because it is strong and stable.

The origin of the muscle is generally fixed and does not move with natural motions. The origin is typically near to the body.

Insertion: A muscle's attachment point that moves when the muscle contracts. Typically, the insertion location is distant.

The belly of the muscle is the bulky or fleshy region of the muscle that participates actively in contraction.

Tendon: A fibrous or connective tissue band that joins the muscle to the bone.

Ligament: A tough fibrous substance that joins bones.

Body Movements

Flexion: A term used to describe the movement of the body during a bending movement.

As a result of flexion, the angle between the two bodily portions is reduced. When you flex your wrist, you are bending your wrist.

Extension: A term used to describe the straightening of a joint. When you stand up, for example, you extend your knee. When you sit, your knees are flexed (bent).

Abduction: A bodily movement that draws an organ away from the body's midline. When you spread your fingers, for example, you are abducting them.

Adduction is the inverse of abduction. The motion of adduction draws the bodily component towards the midline or inwards. You are adducting your fingers when you bring them together.

Rotation: Any movement that rotates a body part is referred to as a rotation. Internal rotation means toward the axis of the body; external rotation means away from the center of the body.

The ankle joint performs foot movements such as dorsiflexion and plantar flexion. *Dorsiflexion* brings the toes near to the shin.

Plantar flexion is the downward movement of the toes. This occurs when you press the brake pedal. A tiptoeing ballerina is plantar flexing.

The rotating movement of the forearm or lower leg is described by the phrases pronation and supination.

Pronate: Rotate downward (when you pronate your arm, the palm faces down)

Supinate: Rotate up (when you supinate your arm the palm faces up)

Eversion and inversion are ankle movements.

Eversion: The sole of the foot slides away from the midline of the body

Inversion: The sole of the foot moves towards the midline of the body

When you tilt your foot, the bottom of your foot slides away from the midline. The sole of the foot moves inwards towards the center during inversion. You invert your foot when you twist it.

Summary

- CMAs need a basic understanding of human anatomy and physiology.
- Anatomy involves studying the structure and formation of the body.
- Physiology refers to the study of how the body works or functions.
- The heart pumps blood throughout the body, with four chambers: atria and ventricles.
- Valves in the heart prevent the backward flow of blood.
- Arteries transport oxygenated blood, while veins return deoxygenated blood.
- The brain controls bodily functions and emotions, with various regions and lobes.
- The pituitary gland produces hormones like vasopressin and oxytocin.
- The autonomic nervous system controls involuntary functions such as breathing.
- The spinal cord has 33 vertebrae, protecting and supplying the body.
- Hormones produced by endocrine glands are essential for growth, development, and balance.
- Examples include ACTH, LH, FSH, insulin, and glucagon.
- The gastrointestinal tract processes food through mechanical and chemical breakdown.
- The liver is vital when it comes to digestion and detoxification.
- The respiratory system switches oxygen and carbon dioxide through organs like the nose, trachea, bronchi, lungs, and alveoli.
- The diaphragm helps with breathing, and the system also enables talking and airway protection.
- The skeletal system includes the axial and appendicular systems, providing protection, support, and mobility.
- Cartilage, tendons, and ligaments have critical roles.
- Conditions like osteoporosis and osteoarthritis are common skeletal issues.
- The urinary system consists of kidneys, which filter waste and balance fluid.
- Nephrons are microscopic filters in the kidneys, and kidney injuries can lead to failure.
- Ureters carry urine from the kidneys to the bladder. The bladder can hold up to two cups of urine.
- Nerves control bladder function and urination, while sphincter muscles prevent leaks.

- The female reproductive system produces and delivers eggs, with internal organs like the vagina, ovaries, and uterus.
- The uterus protects and nurtures a fertilized egg during pregnancy, and fallopian tubes transfer eggs.
- Ovaries produce and store eggs in the female reproductive system.
- The male reproductive system lacks a uterus and ovaries but includes testicles, ducts, and glands.
- Accessory glands produce fluids needed for sperm, and the penis facilitates sperm transfer.
- Testicles produce and store sperm in the male reproductive system.
- The integumentary system is composed of nails, glands, skin, and hair.
- Common skin disorders include dermatitis, melanoma, and shingles.
- Surgical and medical positions vary based on surgery type, anesthesia, and access requirements.
- Patient safety and comfort are crucial during positioning.
- Anatomical terms describe position and movement, such as anterior, posterior, or lateral.
- Planes (sagittal, frontal, transverse) are used to describe anatomical sections.
- Anatomical terms for muscles include origin, insertion, tendons, and ligaments.
- Terms like flexion, extension, abduction, and adduction describe movements.
- Rotation can be internal or external, and pronation and supination refer to forearm or leg rotation.
- Eversion and inversion are ankle movements.

CHAPTER 5
Common Organ Disorders

HUMAN DISEASES FREQUENTLY impact many structures in addition to one or more specific organs. You will need to have a basic understanding of the ailments that could impact particular organs when working as a CMA. CMAs collaborate with physicians who have a variety of specialties. There are those who specialize in treating nervous system problems, and there are people who specialize in treating cardiac problems. Any organ of the body that your doctor treats requires that you know a little bit about its anatomy and pathology.

Areata alopecia: When the hair follicles are attacked, it causes hairfall. The scalp and/or face may develop circular bald spots. Fortunately, recuperation usually occurs spontaneously but can take a few months because the cause is unknown.

Arthritis: This is a general phrase that is frequently used to refer to illnesses that affect the joints. For instance, there is joint swelling and inflammation in osteoarthritis.

Rheumatoid illness: This is systemic, symmetrical in distribution, and affects the tiny joints, is another fairly prevalent ailment.

Autoimmune disorders: Different organs are attacked and damaged by the body's immune system. In other words, your immune system begins to attack your own body cells because it thinks they are alien invaders. Joint swelling, rash, fever, and other medical issues are brought on by the disorder, a classic of which is lupus.

Liver cirrhosis: One of the most prevalent liver conditions is The liver becomes permanently scarred as a result of liver cirrhosis, and there is no prospect of recovery. Alcohol abuse is one of the main contributors to chronic diseases, along with cancer and infections like hepatitis B and C.

Gallstones: They are a condition where the gallbladder produces stones. They could result in anorexia, fever, and pain. The common bile duct can get blocked or even dislodged by the stones. Nowadays, laparoscopic surgery is its treatment of choice.

Hemochromatosis: The disorder known as hemochromatosis is brought on by iron buildup in the liver. Iron buildup in the liver eventually results in serious liver damage. Iron can accumulate in other organs, such as the kidney and pancreas, even though this illness is not very frequent. Most likely, the damaged organ dies as a result of this.

Viral hepatitis: Hepatitis is the medical term for liver inflammation. Viral hepatitis comes in three different forms: A, B, and C. Hepatitis B infection can be avoided with a vaccination.

Liver failure: As the name suggests, liver failure is a condition in which the liver is no longer operating as it should. Liver failure can quickly result in death. The two main causes of liver failure are alcohol and hepatitis C. It might be related to an acetaminophen overdose in kids.

Arrhythmia: A condition in which the heart irregularly beats. It results from modifications to the heart's electrical conduction impulses. Arrhythmias come in many forms, and they can cause unexpected death. The majority of arrhythmias require medical care.

Cardiomyopathy: This disease weakens heart muscles, causing them to lose their ability to pump blood. The patient experiences significant organ and heart failure as a result.

Coronary Artery Disease: This condition is brought on by a buildup of cholesterol and fat on the aortic and arterial walls. The buildup of cholesterol causes artery constriction, which impairs blood flow. A heart attack may result when arteries are fully blocked, which can happen under specific circumstances.

Pericarditis: This occurs when the pericardium is inflamed. The pericardium is the membrane that wraps the heart. This disorder can develop after open heart surgery, viral infections, autoimmune diseases, or other conditions. In most instances, the illness is treatable.

Angina pectoris: A shortage of oxygen to the muscles causes a cardiac ailment known as angina pectoris. Chest pain and perhaps shortness of breath will be experienced by the sufferer. The chest pain disappears after taking the right prescription to widen the blood arteries. However, the patient must visit the closest emergency room if the chest pain doesn't go away.

Asthma: The bronchi, which are the airways, are inflamed, and breathing becomes labored and wheezy as a result of this rather frequently. Numerous things, such as allergic reactions, smoke, dust, pet dander, and smog, may cause this illness. It can be healed with medications and is reversible.

Bronchiectasis: Repeated airway inflammation leads to the condition known as bronchiectasis, which finally causes the lungs and airways to be destroyed. The untreatable condition manifests as shortness of breath, coughing, inability to tolerate physical activity, and significant sputum production.

COPD: A lung condition known as chronic obstructive pulmonary disease (COPD) causes breathing problems because it damages the lungs. Smoking, smog, and lung infections may make it worse.

Cystic fibrosis: Cystic Fibrosis is a rare hereditary disorder that makes clearing mucus from the airways challenging. As a result, there is an excessive buildup of mucus in the airways, which finally causes pneumonia and bronchitis to manifest. It is incurable.

Pleuritis: The medical condition known as pleuritis is brought on by inflammation of the pleura, which lines the lungs. Breathing is painful for those who have pleuritis. Occasionally, infections, autoimmune diseases, and pulmonary embolisms might set off this illness.

Acute renal failure: An illness called acute renal failure is brought on by sick kidneys. The condition could be brought on by acute sickness, pharmaceutical use, or dehydration. When the kidney is not working, the patient typically has elevated test values. The majority of acute cases do improve with the right care, but some could develop into chronic renal failure.

Nephrotic syndrome: Large levels of protein are filtered out of the urine by the kidneys in nephrotic syndrome. Due to the loss of anticoagulation-related proteins, protein loss causes widespread edema and increases the risk of blood clot formation.

Papillary necrosis: Damage to the renal papillae is a symptom of papillary necrosis. It frequently results from the usage of NSAIDs. With supportive care, the condition typically spontaneously improves. However, some people may experience total renal failure and need dialysis.

Pyelonephritis: The illness known as pyelonephritis is brought on by a bladder infection. It is a severe ailment with fever and chills. Urine frequently contains signs of pus, and it urgently needs antibiotic therapy. For pain management and antibiotics, some patients might need to be hospitalized.

Incontinence: Urine spilling is known as incontinence. It is a fairly prevalent issue in society, particularly with the elderly. Prostate enlargement is a typical cause of incontinence in men. There is a persistent want to urinate, and the urine leaks get worse. There are different types of urinary incontinence, and a urologist's consultation is strongly advised because they all require various therapies.

UTI: One of the most typical disorders that impact the urinary system is urinary tract infection (UTI). When bacteria get into the urinary tract, this disease develops. Fever, malaise, frequent urination, painful urination, or urine blood are all possible symptoms. The best way to treat UTIs is with an antibiotic; however, they do have a propensity to come back. Women experience this condition more frequently than men. According to statistics, UTIs affect the average woman at least twice throughout her lifetime.

Interstitial cystitis: Interstitial Cystitis (IC) is a complicated bladder illness that manifests as recurrent spasms. The syndrome is also referred to as painful bladder syndrome. Females are more likely than males to develop interstitial cystitis, which manifests as recurrent abdominal pain, pain in the lower pelvic region, or a pressure-like feeling in the belly. Scarring of the bladder, which eventually reduces its flexibility, is the condition's cause. The bladder cannot contain a lot of urine when it is terrified and unable to expand. As a result of the pressure on the bladder, the patient has persistent pelvic pain.

Ovarian cancer: A rare cancer that affects women is ovarian cancer. It is deadly and cunning. Abdominal distension, bloating, weight loss, back pain, and lower abdominal discomfort are early warning signals. By the time cancer is diagnosed, it has almost always spread because there are no specific symptoms or tests for it. Surgery is the only effective treatment, but chemotherapeutic drugs are used to control it once it has spread. Following ovarian cancer, the overall survival percentage is low.

Menstrual cramping: In young women, menstrual cramping is a highly prevalent condition. This illness causes stomach pain either before or during the menstrual cycle. Although all women may suffer some degree of monthly cramping, others experience really painful cramps. Women who are having monthly periods may have severe discomfort for anywhere between one and six days. People who have severe cramping might need to take medicine to treat the illness.

Vaginal yeast infection: Another typical ailment that affects the female reproductive system, specifically the vagina, is vaginal yeast infection. A yeast fungus develops on the vagina as a result of the disorder. It could spread to the uterus if it is not treated quickly, but this is uncommon. The good news is that using over-the-counter medicine is a simple way to address the illness.

Endometriosis: Endometriosis is a disorder whereby endometrial (the uterine wall) fragments implant in other parts of the body. Infertility and painful periods are all side effects of the illness.

Pelvic inflammatory disease: An infectious condition of the female reproductive organs is referred to as pelvic inflammatory disease. Sexually transmitted diseases (STDs), mainly gonorrhea and chlamydia, are responsible for the disorder. STDs can be dangerous and require medical attention. They can cause female infertility if not treated in a timely manner.

Prostate cancer: A frequent cancer that affects many men is prostate cancer. The prostate gland is enlarged as a result of the cancer, eventually obstructing the flow of urine. Additionally, the patient may experience frequent urination, erectile dysfunction, and blood-stained semen. A rectal exam might find it.

Prostatitis: The enlargement of the prostate gland is a symptom of prostatitis. Urination and ejaculation are frequently uncomfortable in this situation. Additionally, it may result in stomach ache. It is a widespread condition that many guys experience.

Vitiligo: Another skin disorder that causes white patches on the skin. Melanocytes, the skin's pigment-producing cells, are killed in this condition.

Bursitis: Bursitis is a medical disorder that causes some body parts to swell and hurt. It targets the bones and muscles in particular. Fortunately, the illness is easily diagnosable and treatable.

Epidermolysis bullosa: A generic name used to describe a group of illnesses that cause the growth of uncomfortable blisters is epidermolysis bullosa. Blisters are painful by nature, but they tend to appear rather frequently in those who have this ailment.

Pemphigus: Pemphigus: When the immune system attacks the skin's surface, a disease known as pemphigus develops. As a result, the skin's surface becomes injured, resulting in painful blisters.

Psoriatic arthritis: Only those with psoriasis are prone to this type of arthritis. Skin patches that are scaly, white, and red start to appear on the patient. Some of these psoriasis sufferers will eventually develop arthritis, which is quite damaging.

Rheumatoid arthritis: Rheumatoid arthritis is a symmetrical, systemic illness that can impact tiny joints. However, the person may also experience fever, a rash, and heart and lung issues. The most typical symptoms of RA include joint pain, stiffness, and edema. The illness also brings on a very high fever and exhaustion.

Rosacea: Rosacea is a chronic illness that causes pimples and skin redness on the face. Despite the fact that the ailment mostly impacts the skin surrounding the nose and eyes, it is known to cause ocular issues. Long-term persistence of the illness could result in thicker skin.

Spinal stenosis: Spinal stenosis is a condition brought on by the spinal cord's narrowing. The spinal cord's precise dimensions enable the nerves to pass through without being squeezed. When the spine grows too thin, pressure is placed on the nerves, which can result in excruciating back pain.

Sports injuries: Sports accidents can lead to a variety of ailments. Acute and chronic are the different categories. Some sports injuries may fully recover depending on the severity, while others may require lifelong care.

Tendinitis: This ailment results in joint pain and swelling. It happens when the tendon that connects the bone sustains recurrent trauma from either sports- or job-related incidents.

Erectile dysfunction: Males who have erectile dysfunction are unable to achieve or maintain an erection for extended periods of time. According to statistics, one in ten men experience chronic erectile dysfunction. Despite the fact that it is a relatively prevalent ailment, it is rarely discussed because of the stigma attached to it. Erectile dysfunction, however, might only be a sign of a far more serious underlying medical disease. Those with long-term chronic illnesses (e.g., heart disease) are more prone to experience erectile dysfunction.

Summary

- Human diseases impact various structures and organs.
- CMAs need a basic understanding of organ-related ailments.
- CMAs work with specialists in different organ systems.
- Knowledge of organ anatomy and pathology is essential.
- Areata alopecia causes hair loss with circular bald spots.
- Arthritis includes joint swelling and inflammation.
- Rheumatoid Illness is systemic and affects small joints.
- Autoimmune disorders lead to the body attacking its own organs.
- Liver cirrhosis results in permanent scarring.
- Gallstones can cause anorexia, fever, and pain.
- Hemochromatosis is due to iron buildup in the liver.
- Viral hepatitis comes in three forms: A, B, and C.
- Liver failure can be life-threatening.
- Arrhythmia involves irregular heartbeats.
- Cardiomyopathy weakens heart muscles.
- Coronary artery disease results from cholesterol buildup.
- Pericarditis is inflammation of the heart's membrane.
- Angina pectoris causes chest pain.
- Asthma leads to breathing difficulties.
- Bronchiectasis damages the lungs and airways.
- COPD is a lung disease worsened by smoking.
- Cystic fibrosis causes mucus buildup in the airways.
- Pleuritis leads to painful breathing.
- Acute renal failure is due to sick kidneys.
- Nephrotic syndrome involves protein loss in urine.
- Papillary necrosis results from damage to renal papillae.

- Pyelonephritis is a kidney infection.
- Incontinence is urine leakage.
- UTI is a common urinary system infection.
- Interstitial cystitis causes bladder spasms.
- Ovarian cancer is rare but deadly.
- Menstrual cramping leads to stomach pain.
- Vaginal yeast infection is a fungal vaginal infection.
- Endometriosis involves endometrial tissue growth.
- Pelvic inflammatory disease is a female reproductive organ infection.
- Prostate cancer affects the prostate gland.
- Prostatitis causes prostate enlargement and discomfort.
- Vitiligo can lead to white patches on the skin.
- Bursitis leads to swelling and pain in body parts.
- Epidermolysis bullosa causes painful blisters.
- Pemphigus is an autoimmune disease with skin blistering.
- Psoriatic arthritis is linked to psoriasis.
- Rheumatoid arthritis is a systemic joint condition.
- Rosacea causes facial pimples and redness.
- Spinal stenosis is when the spinal cord narrows.
- Sports injuries vary in severity.
- Tendinitis leads to joint pain and swelling.
- Erectile dysfunction means cannot maintain an erection.

CHAPTER 6

ECG

THE ECG IS one of the exams that CMAs run into the most frequently in their line of work. It is among the quickest and simplest examinations to know the patient's cardiac condition. Moreover, the test can be done in a clinic and needs no preparation time. Understanding why, how, and when the ECG should be performed is important because it can save lives.

A non-invasive diagnostic method to examine the electrical pathways of the heart is the electrocardiogram (ECG/EKG). The heart's electrical activity is graphically captured by the ECG.

A medical examination called an ECG is used to evaluate the patient's heart. Electrodes are used in the test, which are applied to the patient's arms, chest, and legs and wired to a device. It's vital to understand that the CMA does not use the ECG to make any kind of diagnosis. The key is understanding how to correctly configure and operate the equipment.

Why Is an ECG Done?

The ECG exam can help in diagnosing the following:

- Myocardial ischemia
- Conduction issues
- Cardiac chamber enlargement
- Determine whether the patient needs a pacemaker by looking for abnormalities in rate and rhythm, such as ventricular fibrillation, premature ventricular contractions, and atrial fibrillation.

Applying the ECG Leads to the Patient

Twelve leads are used to give the ECG exam. Differently angled electrical impulses passing through the heart are captured by each lead.

An ECG can be completed in 5–10 minutes. The setup takes up the majority of the time. Only 10 to 15 seconds are spent actually recording. To prevent artifacts, make sure the patient doesn't move.

Reading an ECG

A doctor interprets the ECG, and the waveforms are examined. Following are the results of measuring the various intervals:

- Rate – the heart rate
- Rhythm – the regularity of the cardiac cycle and evaluates the various intervals.
- Axis – The position and direction of the heart's electrical conductivity
- Hypertrophy – to check whether the atria or ventricles are enlarged
- Ischemia –if the patient is experiencing a heart attack
- Infarction – If the patient has previously experienced a heart attack.

What Happens If the ECG Doesn't Give Enough Information?

Sometimes the ECG may not show any cardiac issues or may not give enough information, but if there is a strong likelihood that a heart ailment exists, other tests can be performed, such as:

Exercise electrocardiography: In order to replicate the symptoms, the heart may occasionally need to be physically stressed. Consequently, the ECG is observed on a screen when the patient works out.

The use of sound waves in an echocardiogram is a non-invasive method for examining the heart valves, cardiac contraction, and the presence of any fluid around the heart.

Holter: Some individuals might have sporadic cardiac rhythms that an ECG might miss. The patient is told to wear a Holter monitor in these situations. Simply said, the patient is placed with a little gadget that continuously records the heart rate for a few days. The device is taken out and examined after the patient returns to the hospital.

Who Does the ECG?

Nurses, medical assistants, doctors, and physician assistants can all do the ECG. Medical assistants frequently do the ECG in clinics.

ECG equipment comes in a variety of forms, and setting them up and understanding how to interpret the heart monitor both require training. Most CMAs receive on-the-job training in ECG and improve their skill over time.

ECG Preparation

Even though preparing for an ECG doesn't take much time, there are still a few things that need to be done, including the following:

1. Positioning the paper in the machine and ensuring that the gain and speed are set in accordance with the doctors' instructions. The standard gain is 100/mV, and the standard speed is 25 mm/sec.
2. Explain to the patient the protocol
3. With patient information, the electrocardiograph is programmed.
4. Take away any and all electrical or electronic items from the patient, including watches and cellphones.
5. Take off any jewelry, including chains and bracelets.
6. The patient should be entirely naked to the ankles.
7. Request that the patient lie face down on the bed.
8. Clean the body parts where the ECG electrodes will be positioned with an alcohol solution.
9. Apply the electrodes to the ankles, chest, and wrist.
10. Advise the patient to remain still and silent throughout the exam.
11. Compute the ECG.
12. Before removing the electrodes from the patient's body, be sure the ECG is what you want.
13. Whenever printing an ECG, always attach a label with the patient's name. Include the test's date and time.

Equipment for an EKG

EKG requires the following supplies:

- Gauze and skin prep solution
- Electrodes
- Razor and tape to remove hair
- Skin adhesive
- ECG paper

Mastering ECGs

Following are examples of pointers to learn and master ECG:

Observe the color: Use the American Heart Association's approved color codes to put the electrodes properly.

Red, yellow, and, green are the three hues that are used, and they are arranged in a clockwise motion.

- Start with the right arm with red
- Move on to the left leg with green
- For the right leg, black

Location of Precordial leads

1. Count the spaces between the ribs. Beginning at the fourth intercostal space (ICS), go along the right edge of the sternum.
2. In the fourth ICS, leads V1 and V2 are positioned on the right and left sides of the sternum.
3. Next, proceed along the fourth ICS and the remaining V-leads (V3 to V6) until you reach the left midclavicular line.
4. V6 is positioned in line with V4 at the fifth ICS, in the midaxillary line.
5. V5 is positioned between V6 and V4 in the anterior axillary at the fifth intercostal gap.

6. V4 is positioned on the midclavicular line at the fifth intercostal gap.

7. V3 is positioned between V2 and V4.

ECG Basics

- The P wave signifies the atrial contraction or depolarization.
- The QRS complex signifies the ventricular contraction or depolarization.
- The T wave indicates the heart's state of rest or repolarization.

Summary

- ECGs are frequently encountered by CMAs in their work, offering a quick and straight-forward way to assess a patient's cardiac health, often requiring no special preparation. Knowing when, why, and how to perform an ECG is essential for potentially life-saving applications.
- An ECG is a non-invasive diagnostic method for examining the heart's electrical pathways, capturing its electrical activity graphically.
- The ECG helps diagnose conditions like myocardial ischemia, conduction issues, cardiac chamber enlargement, and abnormalities in rate and rhythm, such as ventricular fibrillation, premature ventricular contractions, and atrial fibrillation.
- The ECG involves twelve leads to capture different electrical impulses passing through the heart, taking 5–10 minutes to complete with most time spent on setup to prevent patient movement artifacts.
- A doctor interprets the ECG, assessing waveforms and measuring intervals, including rate, rhythm, axis, hypertrophy, ischemia, and infarction.
- When the ECG doesn't provide sufficient information, other tests like exercise electrocardiography, echocardiograms, and Holter monitors may be employed.
- ECGs can be performed by nurses, medical assistants, doctors, and physician assistants, with training and skill development being crucial.
- ECG preparation includes equipment setup, patient explanation, programming, removing electronics from the patient, patient undressing, cleaning electrode areas, applying electrodes, advising patient stillness, computation, label attachment, and equipment and supply management.

- ECG equipment and supplies include gauze, skin prep solution, electrodes, razors, tape, skin adhesive, and ECG paper.
- Mastering ECGs involves following color codes for electrode placement, knowing the locations of precordial leads, and understanding ECG basics: P wave for atrial contraction, QRS complex for ventricular contraction, and T wave for cardiac repolarization.

CHAPTER 7

Medical Terminologies

MEDICAL TERMINOLOGY IS a specific sort of language that is used in the medical field. The language is about the human body and its various illnesses, operations, treatments, and diagnoses. MAs must acquire medical language in order to speak with physicians and patients about health-related issues. Recording patient information and taking vitals are important aspects of their profession, and they must be knowledgeable about the issue. Medical terminology is essential for competent medical coding.

Medical Abbreviations

Medicine, more than any other field, makes extensive use of acronyms. This is because many words are long and difficult to pronounce. As a result, medical professionals use abbreviations to facilitate communication. If you are unfamiliar with common medical abbreviations, you may find your job as a CMA difficult. This guide has all of the abbreviations you need to get started.

ABG Arterial blood gas

AFB Acid fast bacilli

ACL Anterior cruciate ligament

AD Pertaining to the right ear

ADHD Attention deficit hyperactivity disorder

A.Fib Atrial fibrillation

ALS Amyotrophic lateral sclerosis

AMA Against medical advice

AS Pertaining to the left ear

AU Pertaining to both ears

BE Barium enema

BID Twice a day

BUN Blood urea nitrogen

BP Blood pressure

BR Bed rest

BS Bowel sounds or breath sounds

BSO Bilateral salpingo-oophorectomy

Bx Biopsy

C&S Culture and sensitivity

CABG Coronary artery bypass grafting

CAD Coronary artery disease

Cal Calorie

Cath Catheter

CBC Complete blood count

CCU Coronary care unit

CHF Congestive heart failure

CK Creatine kinase

CNA Certified nursing assistant

CNS Central nervous system

COPD Chronic obstructive pulmonary disease

CPAP Continuous positive airway pressure

CPR Cardiopulmonary resuscitation

CRF Chronic renal failure

CRP C-Reactive protein

CSF Cerebrospinal fluid

CT Computerized tomography

CXR Chest X-ray

DC Discharge

DNR Do not resuscitate

DOE Dyspnea on Exertion

Dx Diagnosis

ECC/EKG Electrocardiogram

ED Emergency department

EEG Electroencephalogram

EMG Electromyogram

ENT Ear, nose, throat

ERCP Endoscopic retrograde cholangiopancreatography

ESR Erythrocyte sedimentation rate

FH Family history

FBS Fasting blood sugar

F/u Follow-up

FWB Full weight bearing

Fx Fracture

GB Gallbladder

GCS Glasgow Coma Scale

GERD Gastroesophageal reflux disease

Gest Gestation

GI Gastrointestinal

GSW Gunshot wound

GTT Glucose tolerance test

GYN Gynecology

Hb/HgB Hemoglobin

HB Heart block

HbA1c Glycosylated hemoglobin

HBV Hepatitis B virus

Hct Hematocrit

HDL High-density lipoprotein

H&H Hemoglobin and hematocrit

HIV Human immunodeficiency virus

H/o History of

H&P History and physical

HPS Hantavirus pulmonary syndrome

HR Heart rate

HTN Hypertension

Hx History

IBD Inflammatory bowel disease

ICU Intensive care unit

ICP Intracranial pressure

IDDM Insulin-dependent diabetes mellitus

IM Intramuscular

INR International normalization ratio

I&O Intake and output

IV Intravenous

IVP Intravenous pyelogram

JP Jackson-Pratt drain

K Potassium

KUB X-ray of the kidney, ureters, bladder

Lab Laboratory

LCIS Lobular carcinoma in situ

LDH Lactic dehydrogenase

LDL Low-density lipoprotein

LMP Last menstrual period

LOC Loss of consciousness

LOS Length of stay

LP Lumbar puncture

MTBI Mild traumatic brain injury

MCA Middle cerebral artery

Mets Metastasis

MCH Mean corpuscular hemoglobin

MCV Mean corpuscular volume

MG Myasthenia gravis

Mg Magnesium

MI Myocardial infarction

MICU Medical intensive care unit

MRI Magnetic resonance imaging

MRSA Methicillin-resistant *Staphylococcus aureus*

MVA Motor vehicle accident

Na Sodium

NAD No apparent distress

NC Nasal cannula

NG Nasogastric

NICU Neonatal intensive care unit

NKDA No known drug allergies

NOS Not otherwise specified

NPO Nothing by mouth

NST Non-stress test

N&V Nausea and vomiting

NYD Not yet diagnosed

O2 Oxygen

O2 sat Oxygen saturation

OA Osteoarthritis

OD Right eye

O&P Ova and parasites

OR Operating room

OS Left eye or mouth

OTC Over-the-counter

OU Both eyes

PA Physician's assistant

PACU Post-anesthesia care unit

Pap Pap smear

PAT Paroxysmal atrial tachycardia

Path Pathology

PCA Patient controlled analgesia

PE Physical exam

PE Pulmonary embolism

PED Pediatrics

PET Positron emission tomography

PFT Pulmonary function test

PH Past history

PICC Peripherally inserted central catheter

PICU Pediatric intensive care unit

PID Pelvic inflammatory disease

PMH Past medical history

PRN "as needed"

PRBC Packed red blood cells

PROM Passive range of motion

PSA Prostate-specific antigen

PT Physical therapy

PT Prothrombin time

PTT Partial thromboplastin time

PUD Peptic ulcer disease

PVD Peripheral vascular disease

Q Every

Qhs Every night

Qid Four times per day

RA Rheumatoid arthritis

RBC Red blood cell count

RCA Right coronary artery

RN Registered nurse

R/O Rule out

ROM Range of motion

RT Respiratory therapy

Rx Prescription, therapy

SCD Sudden cardiac death

SCI Spinal cord injury

SGOT Serum glutamic oxaloacetic transaminase

SH Social history

SICU Surgical intensive care unit

SIDS Sudden infant death syndrome

SOB Shortness of breath

STAT Immediately

STD Sexually transmitted disease

Strep Streptococcus

Sx Symptoms

T3 Triiodothyronine

T3 Thyroxine

TB Tuberculosis

TBI Traumatic brain injury

T&C Type and cross

TIA Transient ischemic attack

TID Three times a day

TPN Total parenteral nutrition

TSH Thyroid-stimulating hormone

Tx Treatment

U/A Urinalysis

UGI Upper gastrointestinal series

UO Urinary output

URTI Upper respiratory tract infection

UTI Urinary tract infection

VF Ventricular fibrillation

VS Vital signs

WBAT Weight bearing as tolerated

WBC White blood cell count

WNL Within normal limits

Wt Weight

w/o Without

w/u Workup

Summary

- The importance of medical terminology as a specialized language for healthcare practitioners is emphasized in this chapter.
- Medical Assistants (MAs) must be fluent in medical terminology in order to communicate successfully with physicians and patients.
- Medical terminology is essential for duties such as documenting patient information and taking vital signs.
- The chapter includes a comprehensive collection of medical acronyms that are widely used to simplify difficult phrases and speed up communication.
- For accurate medical coding, mastery of medical abbreviations and terminology is required.

CHAPTER 8

Bloodborne Pathogen Accidents

EVERY PERSON WHO works in a clinical setting, medical lab, healthcare facility, or research facility may come into touch with another person's body fluids, placing them at a high risk of contracting bloodborne diseases. What exactly are bloodborne pathogens?

Bloodborne pathogens are microorganisms transmitted in body fluids that cause diseases in humans. Bloodborne pathogens can be viral, bacterial, and fungal species and are capable of inflicting potentially deadly and severe infections. Being knowledgeable about bloodborne pathogens and using avoidance techniques are essential for staying safe.

Today, 5.6 million healthcare professionals deal in the US regularly with bloodborne viruses, and despite taking all reasonable precautions, a few people contract the disease each year. Adopting the basic infectious disease protocols specified by the CDC and OSHA is one strategy to prevent bloodborne diseases.

Bloodborne Pathogens: What Are They?

Bloodborne pathogens are by definition organisms that cause disease and are easily spread from person to person by contact with bodily fluids like blood. These are some more bodily secretions that might spread pathogens:

- Serum
- Blood
- Semen
- Genital secretions
- Saliva
- Cerebrospinal fluid
- Amniotic fluid
- Pleural, peritoneal, and synovial fluid

Although wearing PPE is strongly advised, saliva, urine, feces, and sweat are generally the least likely to spread germs. In addition to blood, transmission by vaginal fluids or semen is regarded as high risk.

The majority of bloodborne infections spread after coming into contact with blood. The following are typical bloodborne pathogens that are spread through blood:

- HIV
- Hepatitis B, C
- Zika virus
- Malaria
- Ebola virus
- West Nile virus

Hepatitis B, C, and HIV, however, make up the vast majority of bloodborne pathogens in North America.

These infections cause both acute and chronic disorders, characterized by malaise, fever, jaundice, rash, weight loss, anorexia, etc., once they have been acquired. There may be periodic flare-ups of the diseases. There is no vaccination to prevent HIV or hepatitis C, but there is a vaccine for hepatitis B.

The OSHA Bloodborne Pathogens Standard

The guidelines on bloodborne infections were initially released by OSHA (the Occupational Safety And Health Administration) in 1991. According to these recommendations, hospitals and clinics should take proactive measures to reduce worker exposure to bloodborne diseases. The following guidelines are mandated under the OSHA bloodborne standard:

- → Make an exposure control plan and distribute it to all employees. A yearly update of the plan is also required.
- → Reinforce universal safety procedures in the workplace.
- → Ensure that engineering safeguards, such as the availability of self-sheathing needles and sharps disposal bins, are in place.

→ Encourage the use of needle-free techniques whenever possible.

→ Have quick procedures in place for sterilizing and sanitizing the infected or contaminated surface.

→ Ensure that workers reduce the risk of exposure by operating safely.

→ Outfit workers with safety gear, including gloves, masks, gowns, and goggles.

→ All employees should receive a free hepatitis B vaccination, and any infected people should receive a FREE post-exposure examination from an infectious disease expert.

→ There should also be a system in place for reporting any needle stick injuries that result in bloodborne pathogens.

→ Inform staff members on the dangers of bloodborne pathogens, how to properly label specimens, and where to find signage.

Which bodily fluids are subject to universal precautions?

• Cerebrospinal fluid
• Blood
• Semen
• Vaginal discharge
• Synovial fluid
• Fluid from the pericardium and pleura.
• Amniotic fluid

In general, unless they exhibit apparent evidence of infection or contain visible blood, universal precautions do not apply to nasal secretions, feces, perspiration, sputum, urine, or tears.

Who Needs Bloodborne Pathogen Training?

Any person who is susceptible to exposure to bloodborne pathogens, regardless of whether they are a healthcare worker, must complete training and pass the bloodborne pathogens test module. The following professionals should generally be tested for bloodborne pathogens:

First responders, EMTs, paramedics; Firemen and police enforcement; healthcare workers, such as nurses, doctors, phlebotomists, lab techs, etc.; researchers; medical laboratory staff; nursing home employees; dentists and dental assistants; employees of blood banks, cleaning services, and cleaners; school nurses and all other staff members; employees of funeral homes, including morticians; and employees of tattoo parlors.

This list is not exhaustive, but in general, the bloodborne pathogen module test should be administered to everybody who might come into contact with bodily fluids or blood products.

Post-Exposure Treatment

Even with the utmost care and strict adherence to safety measures, incidental contact with bloodborne infections does happen. According to data, nurses and medical professionals will experience a needle poke at least once in their lifetime. A needle or sharp injury will happen to a member of the medical staff at some point throughout their employment if they work in the operating room or emergency department.

The most important thing is to move fast once you have been exposed to bloodborne infections. There should be a post-exposure protocol in place at every business in North America. All companies must provide free post-exposure and follow-up appointments to their staff members who have been hurt by needles, per OSHA regulations.

1. The first thing to do after a needlestick or other sharp injury is to promptly wash the affected area with soap and water. If the mucus barrier has been affected by blood or bodily fluid, use water or saline. Render not less than 10 to 15 minutes doing this.
2. After the initial cleaning, go right away to the emergency room or the workplace occupational and health safety department to get medical help.
3. Ensure that all information regarding your injuries is recorded following company policy.

Your baseline blood work will be performed to ascertain your hepatitis B, C, and HIV status, depending on the seriousness of your needlestick injury and/or contact with the mucosal membranes. Your level of hepatitis B immunity will also be determined by the blood test results.

Treatment

Hepatitis B: If you have already received a hepatitis B vaccination, no further treatment is necessary. If you have never gotten the hepatitis B vaccine or do not have immunity to the disease you will be provided hepatitis B immune globulin and begin receiving the hepatitis B vaccine.

Hepatitis C: There is currently no vaccination to treat hepatitis C, but recently, some highly potent medications have been created that can stop the disease's growth and even provide a cure. The length of the treatment, however, can range from 1 to 6 months.

Tetanus: Even though tetanus is not a bloodborne infection, if the wound has broken the skin, you will be questioned about your tetanus status. Tetanus vaccination is typically advised for deep wounds or wounds caused by filthy materials. If it has been more than ten years since your tetanus injection, a booster is advised for only minor injuries. If the patient received their last booster shot more than five years ago, a booster injection is advised if the wound was brought on by a dirty needle or a deep puncture wound.

Medical facilities need to dress appropriately and uphold strict sanitary standards. Surfaces need to be periodically cleaned and sanitized. Medical waste disposal regulations must be followed while disposing of lab and ward equipment. Regularly used items must always be cleaned and disinfected before use. Infections are prevented by these strict hygiene requirements. Patients should be kept apart from those with extremely contagious illnesses.

Safety Education

Medical facility management should offer, assist, or support safety education in order to keep employees safe. To instruct staff members on how to protect themselves from the aforementioned accidents, facilities could contact safety specialists.

Being proactive and placing a strong emphasis on patient safety is one of the finest strategies to guarantee the facility's safety plan. Patients frequently cause the majority of mishaps that happen in medical facilities. Many issues can arise if a patient gets lost and ends up in a private space like a lab. Educating patients about the various safety measures can help to keep the entire facility safe.

While it can be difficult at times to encourage patients to pay attention to safety precautions, nurses, doctors, and other medical professionals can help the situation. Patients should be politely informed of the safety precautions. Patients will adhere to established recommendations if they receive frequent reminders about places to avoid, things not to do, and other important information.

How to Prevent Accidents at Work

There are three basic sorts of accidents that could happen to the medical staff. To avoid these mishaps, proper planning and security must be taken. Bloodborne pathogens and infections, accidents in radiation rooms, and physical accidents are the three main accidents. Slips and falls, unintentional cuts, and similar events are examples of physical accidents. Physical accidents are typically considered while designing and outfitting medical facilities. For instance, uneven floors increase friction and discourage falling. The medical professional does have a part to play in averting such mishaps, though. Physical mishaps can be avoided if sharp things are handled and stored safely.

Safety Management Systems

Every healthcare facility needs a safety and emergency response strategy. The actions to take in the event of a workplace accident are provided by the safety management system. Three essential elements must be present in every good safety and health management system. These include:

- Accident prevention
- Accident management
- Accident recovery

To strive to reduce accidents, the aforementioned accident prevention strategies ought to be sufficient. Among other things, putting safety measures in place and educating patients and employees could help prevent mishaps.

You must know what to do during accidents in terms of accident management. There are procedures to follow in case of an accident in medical spaces like labs, theaters, and wards. If there is bleeding as a result of an injury, the professional must halt all work until the bleeding has been stopped. If they were handling a crucial task, another medical professional should step in right away. First aid supplies with the ability to stop bleeding must always be present in medical spaces. Such actions can lessen the consequences of an accident at the medical facility. Always don PPE prior to helping a patient who is bleeding or secreting other bodily fluids.

There are a lot of post-accident actions that can be done. The post-accident response could involve assessing the safety precautions that are currently in place, identifying responsible parties, and compensating the harmed parties. The specifics of post-accident actions, however, mostly depend on the type and nature of accident and loss experienced during the process. Always follow your facility's policies and procedures.

First-Aid Emergencies

When you are a CMA working in a medical facility, you are the first person people will call in an emergency. Whether the incident occurs inside the hospital or outside and the patient is brought inside, you must be prepared. There are advised first aid delivery methods. When a patient is in danger and needs emergency care but there is no doctor nearby, first aid can help save the patient's life. But you shouldn't just start administering first aid without following the correct procedure. Below are the steps to follow:

1. Check for potential danger in the area: It's likely that the cause of a person's damage if it appears to be physical, poses a threat to your life as well. Make sure you thoroughly examine the scene to determine safety before you rush in to begin providing first aid. Only when the patient is still at the accident scene does this apply. Let's say the patient was rushed to your hospital. In that instance, if a doctor is not present, you may continue with first aid.

2. Request medical assistance: Before you go to your patient and start to help, be sure you have requested assistance. Make sure you have alerted the doctor of the emergency if one is available, even if they are not present. If you are far from a hospital, call an ambulance right away to send help to the scene while you tend to your patient.

3. Provide care for the patient: After contacting a medical professional or other facility, start helping the patient. While certain medical emergencies lend themselves to first-aid remedies, others do not. Among the situations that require first assistance are minor wounds like:

- o Nasal congestion
- o Burns
- o Sore throats
- o Fever
- o Minor cuts
- o Splinters,
- o Sprains
- o Stings
- o Cough
- o Abrasions

Do not hurry into executing a first aid procedure you are unfamiliar with, even when such conditions are open to first aid care. You should be familiar with standard first aid procedures if you work in healthcare. Additionally, you ought to keep a first aid bag with some of the essential supplies close at hand.

A medical kit's main first aid supplies are as follows:

- Different size band-aids
- Safety pins
- Disposable sterile gloves
- A pair of scissors
- Eye Dressing
- Distilled water
- Triangular bandages
- Painkillers
- Oral decongestants
- Antihistamine pills or cream
- Adhesive tape
- Antacids
- A lighter

Allergy Medication

These are the must-have most frequent components of a first aid kit. With asthma, stomach acids, nasal congestion, fever, and other common illnesses, this kit can aid in stabilizing the patient.

How to Handle Common Emergencies that Require First Aid

If you are unsure of what you are doing, avoid attempting first aid on anyone-seek assistance from someone trained to handle that situation. Most individuals try to administer first aid in a hurry, which only makes things worse. The majority of common diseases can be easily treated by adhering to first aid protocols. These circumstances are as follows:

Choking

Choking is one of the most common accidents that may require first aid assistance. A person will choke when a foreign object, mostly food particles, blocks the air pipe. When this happens, a person cannot breathe, and some signs may occur. Among the common signs of choking include difficulty in talking, difficulty in breathing, unconsciousness, pale or green skin, and shaking. When you spot someone showing any of these signs at the table during a meal, chances are that they are choking and need immediate assistance.

If the patient is still coughing, allow them to continue to get the piece out. If they are unable to cough start the Heimlich maneuver. It is no longer recommended to do a blind finger sweep—only insert your fingers into the victim's mouth if you can clearly see the object and can grab it—if not you could risk logging it further into the airway.

Giving back blows

Attempting back blows without following the right guidelines will only hurt the victim. For an adult, bend the patient at the waist and give five blows with the heel of your hand. Target the shoulder blades to exert force on the chest and push out the piece. For a child, place and bend him or her down on your knees and do the same, but use moderate force considering the child's age. This technique will be demonstrated in your BLS training.

You may also give the patient five abdominal thrusts or alternate between the abdominal thrusts and back blows until the piece gets out.

Bleeding

Bleeding is another emergency situation that may require your response. In the case of excessive bleeding, it is crucial to control the bleeding promptly. Although there are various reasons why people bleed, physical harm is the main reason. Depending on the type and severity of the damage, you should decide whether to administer first aid or not. The best course of action when a wound is extremely bad is to just try to stop or slow the bleeding. Again don PPE to prevent transmission of blood-borne pathogens.

There are various sorts of bleeding besides injury that aren't always brought on by a physical wound. When handling such situations, you ought to exercise a little extra caution. For instance, you need to be careful not to make the patient's bleeding worse if you encounter one who has a nosebleed or vaginal bleeding.

There are specific actions you must take to stop or lessen bleeding while dealing with a patient who is bleeding. The actions conducted should adhere to accepted protocols. The steps to halt external bleeding brought on by physical injury are listed below.

If gloves or other protective equipment is available, wear them to avoid coming into touch with anyone else's bodily fluids.

Apply a clean piece of cloth to the cut and gradually tighten it to stop the blood flow. Hold pressure until the bleeding stops, keep wrapping over the wound.

Do not attempt to remove the cloth or wipe it up if blood is soaked into it. Instead, pile on extra layers of cloth until the wound's blood clots.

Elevate the damaged arm or leg above the heart to reduce bleeding and promote blood clotting over the wound.

After applying the cloth, carefully wash your hands before rushing the patient to the hospital for additional examinations.

Cleanse the wound with a piece of cotton wool immersed in an antiseptic solution, such as surgical spirit, if the bleeding is minimal and may be removed by washing. Cover the wound with a medicated adhesive bandage once it has been cleaned. For injuries that don't require a higher level of treatment, this ought to work.

Other types of bleeding, such as bleeding from the nose, should be treated according to the recommended first aid steps in that situation. Here are the procedures to follow in the event of nose bleeding.

How to stop a bleeding nose

Letting the patient lean forward while sitting erect is important. The blood should be able to softly drop off and onto the ground as a result.

The bleeding should cease and the blood should naturally clot after one to two minutes. Don't let your patient pick their nose, though. Picking the nose could cause it to bleed again, making the condition even worse.

Cold Exposure

A person may sustain serious injuries when exposed longer to the cold. If the body temperature falls below freezing, hypothermia and severe frostbite injuries may result. In that situation, a person can lose their capacity for function and possibly lose a limb or their life. The treatment of hypothermia is urgent since it is a medical emergency. Frostbite is another consequence of exposure to cold. When the body's cells are exposed to the cold for too long, it can result in frostbite.

Frostbite and hypothermia both require prompt medical intervention to avoid amputation or loss of life. It is advised to warm up gradually in cases of hypothermia. Don't rush to warm the patient up with heated towels or showers. Such abrupt temperature swings may cause additional problems.

The patient should ideally be kept in a warm location for some time while being wrapped in warm sheets or garments.

In terms of the proper method, frostbite is similar. Do not immediately immerse the injured region in warm water. Instantaneous heating will only make the situation worse. Do not use hot pads or massage the patient's arms or legs to warm them up. Additionally, you shouldn't give the patient alcohol or cigarettes to warm up quickly. As an alternative, simply keep them warm to aid in bringing their body temperature back to normal.

Asthma Attack

Attacks of asthma are brought on by constriction of the bronchial tube lining. Breathing problems are frequently brought on by the swelling and inflammation of bronchial tubes. If they are not treated right away, they could result in death. Take these actions to aid someone having an asthma attack.

Inquire about the patient's asthma strategy and adhere to the instructions given. The following procedures may be taken if the person does not have an asthma action plan.

Depending on the sort of clothing they are wearing, prop the patient up and adjust or remove their garments.

Help the patient use their inhaler or medication. Most asthmatics carry an inhaler with them at all times. If you have one in your first aid box, you can use it. If not, buying one or switching to an asthma medication is advised.

As soon as the patient begins breathing normally and regains consciousness, assist them. The patient has not improved just because the wheezing ceases. Additionally, you must never abandon a patient who is worn out.

It is very advised to transfer to an emergency room right away.

Insect Bite and Animal Bites

Insect bites can be harmful, therefore they need to be treated carefully. Spiders and snakes, among other insects and animals, can be poisonous. While others, like bees, might cause the sufferer considerable physical harm. In an emergency, treating an insect bite could save a life. The majority of the time, places where medical services are far away are where insect bites happen. If you happen to be there, you might be able to save the patient's life. Common indications of an insect bite include:

- Swelling
- Itchiness
- Redness of the skin
- Vomiting
- Abdominal cramps
- Shock
- Difficulty in breathing
- Swelling of the lips

Perform an emergency first aid procedure for insect bites if you are in a remote area with a patient who has been bitten.

Helping a person stung by an insect

Try to extract the stinger if the insect left one embedded in the flesh. Avoid attempting to remove it with your nails or tweezers. To remove the stinger, simply brush a flat object over the skin where it is buried.

Wash the area with soap and water once the stinger has been removed.

To reduce pain, compress the affected area with clothing or wrap it in an ice bag.

Make a paste by mixing water and baking soda and apply it to soothe painful insect bites like wasp and bee stings.

The insect sting may be extremely deadly and likely to cause death in some circumstances. Send the patient as quickly as possible to the closest institution if you find that they are having trouble breathing, have swollen lips or bodies, or are exhibiting other serious symptoms. First, try to halt the blood flow from the bitten site to the rest of the body for highly toxic bites like a snake bite. If the snakebite is on the leg, the patient should be sent to the closest medical institution for treatment while a piece of cloth should be tightly wrapped above and below the bite.

Seizures

Seizures are frequently handled as emergencies. Even if the individual having seizures has epilepsy, you shouldn't panic. Seizures in people with epilepsy often last between three seconds and two minutes. Convulsions, lip-smacking, loss of awareness, bewilderment, muscle contractions, and convulsions are typical symptoms of seizures.

You could do a few things to assist the patient if you are around someone who is having seizures. The following are some suggested actions: Loosen their clothing and anything else that might restrain the patient; Do not hold them down; Do not put anything in the patient's mouth; Do not hold the patient's tongue; Assist by removing anything dangerous nearby, so the patient does not get hurt.

If at all feasible, support the patient's head on a smooth, flat surface.

Lay the patient on the side to facilitate easy breathing when the seizure has subsided.

Cardiac Arrest

A cardiac arrest occurs when a person's heart suddenly stops beating. It happens when the heart experiences abnormalities in electrical charge. There should be an instant reaction to safeguard the patient from any threats when they experience cardiac arrest. If not properly treated, a cardiac arrest can be fatal even in just minutes. However, administering first assistance could help the patient remain alive.

Unresponsiveness, sweating, shortness of breath, and a drop in heart rate are among the symptoms of cardiac arrest to watch out for. The following actions could be taken if you detect that someone has abruptly stopped breathing and beating their heart:

To assist in reviving the heartbeat, begin CPR right away.

You must perform a CPR count of between 100 and 120 chest compressions per minute to keep the patient alive. A helpful hint to perform CPR at this rate is to sing the song "Staying Alive" in your head and match the compressions to the beat of the song.

Use the external defibrillator in your first aid kit if you have one to attempt to shock the heart back into rhythm.

Continue CPR while waiting for emergency assistance. Before you begin CPR, make sure you dial an emergency number.

Physical Accidents

Physical accidents are another common emergency that CMAs have to handle. These could include everything from business and sports injuries to auto accidents. When there isn't a local medical institution, these accidents also require prompt action. Several different first aid procedures can be used to manage this kind of emergency. Depending on the body part affected and how it happened, a different routine will be used.

Joint Dislocation

Joint dislocation is possible in the event of an accident, whether it be a sports injury or a traffic accident. The elbows, wrists, ankles, and knees are joints that can easily be dislocated. Your course of action should be dictated by your best assessment of the circumstance. If you suspect -stabilize the affected extremity and hasten the patient to an area hospital.

Minor Injuries

Use the RICE method for the first 48 hours when treating minor injuries. RICE is the acronym for rest, ice, compression, and elevation.

Simply rest and apply ice to the joint on the first day. Tighten the joint with a piece of clothing to ease the damaged area, but avoid doing so excessively.

If you have joint discomfort in your arms or legs, raise them above your heart to reduce swelling and promote speedy healing.

A qualified doctor must treat the patient if the pain continues after 48 hours.

Emergency Identification and Response

CMAs are frequently entrusted with responding to emergencies. As a CMA, you must understand what an emergency entails and be ready to react accordingly. If it is determined that your actions did not adhere to professional standards or that you did not give the proper instructions, you can be held accountable for a life lost in an emergency. Always put what you know into practice since a lot of emergencies can happen. Call for aid if you are unsure how to assist.

Top advice for effectively handling emergencies:

1. Don't freak out: If you find yourself in a situation where you need to act quickly, you should strive to remain calm. Given that the situation is urgent, doing this is not a simple task. The goal of your activities, as a medical professional, should be to save as many lives as you can. Only when you are calmly collected can you save the most lives. Stress can cause you to make terrible decisions that you will later regret.
2. Scan the Area for Potential Danger: The next action you should take is to scan the area for any potential threats to your safety. Just because something is urgent doesn't mean you should act immediately. Ensure to not put your life in danger by failing to take the essential precautions if you are at an accident site.

3. Inspect for Bleeding: As soon as you're certain the region is secure, concentrate on taking care of the patient or patients. Start by keeping an eye out for blood. Follow the step continuously if there is no blood. Try to halt the bleeding if any blood is present. Keep in mind, among other things, the principles of justice and nonmaleficence when managing several patients. All the patients should receive your attention, but the more seriously damaged ones should come first.

4. Loosen Clothing: You won't always need to take off your patient's clothes during an emergency. But in the majority of accidents, clothing might make it harder to provide effective first aid. In rare circumstances, a patient's clothing may restrict them, making a full recovery impossible. The best way out is to loosen the patient's garments when they have lost consciousness, have a heart attack or cardiac arrest, or are having seizures. Your ability to care for the patient is much improved by allowing them to take off their garments.

5. Call for Help: If you are outside of a medical facility, contact for assistance before proceeding. Call 911 or any other emergency number where you are confident you can receive prompt assistance. The patient should be picked up by an ambulance ASAP. You must make a call for this to be accomplished. Keep in mind that all of your efforts to assist the patient are limited to first aid. The patient cannot receive care at home at the scene of the accident.

6. Do not move the patient: It is not advisable to move the patient before a medical professional arrives. When there is no other option, just relocate the sufferer. The best course of action would be to move the patient if they had fallen on a highway while having a seizure. If challenged by immediate hazards, like heavy traffic, do not relocate the patient. Check the patient's body while they are still lying down to see whether they have any fractures. Note this information since the doctor may find it useful when they arrive.

7. Perform CPR When Required: As a CMA, you should be familiar with both how to perform CPR and when it is necessary. Many circumstances may lead you to do CPR, but two of them are most typical: when someone's breathing has ceased or when their heart stopped. You can provide CPR in each case to assist the patient in regaining normal bodily functions.

These are some of the initial actions you ought to take in an emergency. There are various emergencies, and maintaining your composure is crucial. You can be confident that you'll act appropriately to provide the patient with the best care just by controlling your panic. The most crucial thing to keep in mind is that you must always preserve professional ethics.

Summary

- Bloodborne pathogens are organisms that cause disease and can be transmitted by bodily fluids such as blood, serum, sperm, vaginal secretions, and others.
- HIV, Hepatitis B and C, Zika virus, Malaria, Ebola virus, and West Nile virus are all common bloodborne infections.
- The most common bloodborne infections in North America are hepatitis B, C, and HIV.
- The OSHA Bloodborne Pathogens Standard (Occupational Safety and Health Administration) establishes rules for preventing worker exposure to bloodborne infections.
- Employees should be vaccinated against hepatitis B, and post-exposure examinations are required for those who have been exposed to bloodborne infections.
- Certain biological fluids, such as cerebral fluid, blood, sperm, vaginal discharge, synovial fluid, and fluids from the pericardium and pleura, are subject to universal precautions.
- Anyone who may be exposed to bloodborne infections, such as healthcare personnel, first responders, researchers, and employees in a variety of sectors, should be trained and tested for bloodborne pathogens.
- Post-exposure strategies are critical for employees who may be exposed to bloodborne pathogens despite safety precautions.
- Following bloodborne pathogen contact, immediate washing of the exposed area, medical treatment, and blood tests are critical.
- Treatment varies based on the pathogen and includes hepatitis B immunization as well as hepatitis C and tetanus treatments.
- To avoid infections in medical institutions, strict hygiene requirements, cleaning, and sanitation are required.
- Patients suffering from contagious disorders should be kept apart from others.
- Employee and patient safety education is critical to maintaining a safe environment.
- Patients should be taught the need for safety precautions.
- Choking: Recognize the signs of choking and administer appropriate back strikes to adults and children.
- Control bleeding by providing pressure to the affected area, elevating it, and cleansing the wound.
- You can cure hypothermia through gradual warming of the patient.

- Asthma Attack: Assist patients in utilizing their inhaler or medication and, if necessary, seek emergency care.
- Insect and animal bites: Remove stingers, clean the area, and seek medical assistance if the reaction is severe.
- Seizures: Make sure the patient is safe, shield their head, and position them on their side.
- Cardiac arrest: Begin CPR immediately and, if accessible, use an external defibrillator.
- Joint Dislocation: For small dislocations, use the RICE (Rest, Ice, Compression, Elevation) treatment; for severe cases, seek medical attention.
- Maintain your cool and examine the situation for potential hazards.
- Check for blood and, if required, loosen clothing.
- For expert medical assistance, contact emergency services.
- If at all possible, avoid moving the patient.
- When CPR is required, perform it.

CHAPTER 9

Hand Hygiene, Sanitizing, Disinfecting, And Sterilization

REGULAR HAND WASHING is one extremely efficient way to stop the spread of healthcare-associated infections to patients and employees.

Teaching healthcare professionals the value of hand washing is one of the fastest ways to save lives every year, according to a wealth of evidence. Each year, one or more nosocomial infections account for 10% to 25% of hospital admissions. Furthermore, the fact that many of the infections are resistant to treatment is worrisome. Both hospitals and local communities are experiencing an increase in antibiotic-resistant pathogens. An estimated one-third of hospitalized patients develop illnesses as a result of contaminated surfaces brought about by frequently contaminated or unwashed hands. Not using sterile gloves and touching sterile materials is one of the most frequent ways to introduce bacteria during compounding in a pharmacy. As a result, hand washing is now expected in all healthcare facilities to assist in lowering the number of infectious bacteria.

As a cost-effective method of minimizing and preventing illnesses, hand washing methods now include routine training and instruction for personnel.

When entering the clinic and before making contact with any patients, hand cleaning is typically done. Before handling drugs and compounding, hand cleansing has become customary.

Hand washing is done prior to and following the administration of the flu vaccine and other vaccinations now that licensed medical assistants are engaged.

Hand Washing Solutions

The following are appropriate hand-cleaning options:

1. Alcohol-based rubs with a 50–90% alcohol content
2. Use plain soap and water, particularly if the hands are visibly soiled

The following are the general guidelines for washing your hands with soap and water:

- Hands should be lathered up with enough soap and washed.
- The wrist creases, palms, webspace between fingers, fingertips, backs of hands, thumb, and fingers are some areas of the hand that need to be cleaned.
- Hands should be washed for at least 15 seconds and then rinsed under warm, running water.
- Hands can then be dried by air or with disposable paper towels.
  1. Use of antibacterial soap under certain conditions
  2. Hand sanitizer wipes are only utilized in the absence of running water and sinks.

The date of expiration is clearly marked on the product containers, so hand hygiene products are not used after that date.

In today's healthcare facilities, wall-mounted hand hygiene dispensers are installed in spaces that have been specifically designated for them, such as the area for preparing medications, the customer counter, the staff room, the computer room, and the bathrooms. For everyone, including clients, patients, and employees, it's crucial to have hand sanitizers or dispensers on hand.

Employees who are unable to properly wash their hands should not be allowed to work in environments that require sterility. Employees with weaning casts or splints, bandages, artificial nails, nail enhancements, hand jewelry, or those who have a severe allergic reaction to the hand washing solutions, in general, are unable to maintain proper hand hygiene.

Hand Washing Frequency

According to need, handwashing frequency varies. While critical care nurses wash their hands 15-20 times each hour on average, regular floor nurses only do so 4–8 times an hour. When assisting with minor procedures or helping to prepare medications, medical assistants must always maintain sterility. They must wash their hands before entering and after leaving the aseptic area.

Factors Affecting Compliance

The original 1975 handwashing recommendations from the Centers for Disease Control and Prevention (CDC) were revised in 1995 and 2002. Despite the significance of hand washing, most healthcare professionals do it less frequently than is advised, and even worse, 5–10% of employees fail to comply at all.

How Long Should One Wash Hands?

The CDC recommends a 15-second hand wash for effective infection management. However, pharmacists who use aseptic procedures like compounding should wash their hands for 30 seconds. Overall, it has been noted that healthcare professionals typically "rinse and run" for 10 seconds.

Sanitizing, Disinfecting, and Sterilization

Sanitizing, disinfecting, and sterilizing are concepts that should be understood by everyone who works in the healthcare industry. Despite the fact that many people use these phrases interchangeably, there are some distinctions between them, thus it is important to understand both their differences and similarities.

What Is Cleaning?

Sanitation or decontamination is different from cleaning. While decontamination involves neutralizing or removing a harmful or toxic substance, radiation, or germs from an object, location, or person, cleaning mostly focuses on removing dust and grime.

Cleaning frequently comes before sanitization or disinfection even when it doesn't actually kill bacteria. This makes disinfection and sanitization more successful. However, disinfection usually comes after cleaning. For instance, after a blood stain on the floor, the stain is first wiped with a wet mop, then a disinfectant is applied.

Sanitization

Most often, sanitizing eliminates or drastically decreases bacteria by at least 99.9%. It is a method of washing, cleaning, or getting rid of dirt or germs on an inanimate surface. It's crucial to realize that sanitization reduces the amount of bacteria by eliminating them rather than killing them, which lowers the likelihood of an infection spreading.

Sanitation is typically performed on surfaces that are not frequently exposed to very dangerous germs. Toys for kids and kitchen utensils, for instance, are perfect for sanitization.

The product must eliminate at least 99.9% of bacteria in order to qualify as a sanitizer. The lower-strength solution of bleach is regarded as a sanitizer, whilst the greater-strength solution is regarded as a disinfectant.

Disinfection

A disinfectant is a substance that kills more than 99.99% of surface-residing bacteria. A disinfectant, as opposed to a sanitizer, will eliminate the bacteria on a surface. There are different clinical applications despite this slight distinction.

For instance, you would use a sanitizer rather than a disinfectant to remove germs from your hands. Inanimate things like the floor, toilet seats, urinals, patient beds, clinic surfaces, etc. are more commonly treated with disinfectants than living ones. A household bleach that contains sodium hypochlorite will kill nearly 100% of the bacteria, in contrast to the majority of alcohol-based hand sanitizers that only kill 99% of hazardous microbes.

Sterilization

While sterilization will kill everything and effectively eliminate all organisms—both good and bad—sanitization and disinfection both focus primarily on germs that are regarded to be harmful. Chemical or physical procedures can be used to disinfect an area. When the work surface where compounding is done has become polluted, for instance, this is a classic example of disinfection in a pharmacy. A solution of formaldehyde, glutaraldehyde, or hydrogen peroxide can be used to clean the surface. It can be essential to leave the product on the surface for 20 minutes or for 12 hours, depending on the disinfectant kind. The traditional method of physical sterilizing involves heating surgical equipment to 200C for 30 minutes in an autoclave.

You won't likely come across any microbes on the pharmacy drug processing surface if you are told that it is sterile.

Common methods of sterilization are as follows:

- o Advanced filtration
- o Dry heat cabinets are usually used for surgical and medical instruments
- o Ethylene oxide gas
- o Hydrogen peroxide gas
- o Ionizing radiation is usually used for medical and surgical instruments and equipment
- o Infrared radiation
- o Heated pressurized steam

Tips for Safe Disinfection

1. To find out if a product is a true disinfectant, read the label. Manufacturers are required by law to mention that on the product label.
2. To find out what kinds of bacteria, fungi, or viruses the disinfectant will kill, read the label. If you're attempting to fight the coronavirus in the office, this is crucial.
3. Avoid mixing different chemicals together; for example, don't use alcohol, hydrogen peroxide, or bleach together; this usually endangers the person using the product more.
4. Whenever working with disinfectants, always use gloves.
5. To find out how long you can leave the solution on the surface, always read the label. Frequently, the label will specify when it is necessary to wipe the surface in order to eliminate the disinfectant.
6. Keep all sanitizers and disinfectants out of the reach of youngsters and in a secure location.

How frequently do you employ these remedies?

Disinfectants are used according to the sort of work being done and the environmental circumstances. If your compounding workplace is constantly unclean, it might need to be cleaned after each action. For instance, the floors and restrooms might need to be disinfected regularly.

Summary

- Hand washing is a critical practice in healthcare to prevent healthcare-associated infections.
- Compliance with proper hand hygiene is essential for patient and staff safety.
- Hand washing should be done before patient contact, medication handling, and after leaving aseptic areas.
- Proper hand washing involves lathering hands with soap, cleaning various hand areas, washing for at least 15 seconds, rinsing with warm water, and drying with air or disposable towels.
- Hand sanitizers and wipes are suitable alternatives when sinks are unavailable.
- Hand lotions can be used after hand washing.
- Hand washing frequency varies based on healthcare roles and tasks.
- In aseptic environments like medication preparation, medical assistants must wash their hands prior to entering and after leaving.
- Sanitization reduces bacteria by at least 99.9% and is used for surfaces with lower germ exposure.
- Disinfection kills more than 99.99% of surface bacteria and is commonly used for surfaces like patient beds.
- Sterilization eliminates all organisms and is typically used for surgical equipment.

CHAPTER 10

Understanding Infection Control

INFECTIOUS AGENTS ARE the carriers of infections. The typical infectious agents include bacteria, fungi, and viruses. Measures used to impede or stop the transmission of infectious pathogens are referred to as infection control. There are a number of ways infectious agents can spread. For example, airborne illnesses spread more quickly and are significantly more challenging to manage.

On the other hand, some illnesses (such as superficial fungal infections) can only be contracted through skin contact. The method employed to control infections also depends on the kind of infection that is present in a certain area. Certain infections require prompt treatment. On the other hand, certain infections can be managed without the need for extensive intervention.

CMAs are crucial linkages in stopping the transmission of infection within a medical facility. Because of this, CMAs are required to have a fundamental knowledge of the different infectious agents and how to manage infections when they manifest.

How to Prevent Infections

Infections must be controlled for a variety of reasons, including the following:

1. To lessen the financial burden: Experts in infectious diseases strive to keep the cost of treating or managing any infectious ailment from rising. Any household, or even the government, can suffer from the costs associated with disease treatment. Only a few people experience infections while they are under control. The cost of treating the patients is consequently decreased.
2. To Decrease Deaths: Some infections are deadly and can quickly cause a large number of deaths. The reduction of mortality is the ultimate goal of infection control. As soon as highly lethal conditions are discovered in a specific area, they must be prevented from spreading. Covid-19 is a prime illustration.
3. Lessening the Demand on Medical Facilities In order to relieve some of the strain on healthcare institutions, it is crucial to control infections. There may be a surge in individ-

uals visiting urgent care centers and emergency rooms when numerous people have the same ailment. If the illnesses are not under control, such a patient influx might cause the health system in a region or a nation to completely collapse.

How to Control Infections

Health facilities, governmental organizations, and experts in infectious diseases use a variety of infection control techniques. Collaboration between CMAs, physicians, and decision-makers is crucial for infection control. Among the techniques used to prevent infections are:

1. Isolation: In the majority of medical facilities, isolation is a strategy for preventing the spread of seriously contagious diseases. For instance, isolating a patient who has an airborne illness that is highly contagious (like active tuberculosis) is the greatest strategy to prevent the illness from spreading to other patients. Even though this method is frequently harshly condemned, there are circumstances when isolating patients is vital.

2. Mass vaccination is a tried-and-true technique for preventing infection. Health professionals advise immunization to prevent the spread of infectious diseases such as the highly contagious coronavirus and measles. When a person receives a vaccination against an infectious disease, they also lower their likelihood of contracting a severe illness from the same infection.

3. Public health education: Raising public awareness is one of the best approaches to combat infection control. It is the responsibility of health professionals to notify the general population of what to do when a highly contagious illness outbreak occurs. Additionally, health professionals must instruct the general public on how to handle infectious specimens (such as sputum and urine) and keep them away from infected people. The use of masks and hand washing are further precautions.

4. Personal Hygiene: Although it doesn't work for all illnesses, personal hygiene is a strategy that some infections respond well to. It is particularly crucial in the battle against viral and bacterial infections. Cleaning hands and maintaining good standards of personal hygiene might help reduce the transmission of an infection (such as cholera influenza) when it is being spread quickly by a specific bacterial infection (such as cholera).

5. Governmental regulations: Finally, laws and regulations issued by the government may aid in halting the spread of diseases. As an illustration, the recommendations given by

numerous nations during the height of COVID-19 were crucial in preventing the illness from spreading. For instance, several nations were largely spared from the development of widespread infection among the local population by the prohibition of incoming passengers from afflicted countries. While government regulations offer a solid foundation for preventing diseases, they can also be abused to restrict the privileges and rights that every person is entitled to.

Although there are numerous elements that affect infection control, medical professionals are ultimately responsible for it. You must be conscious of the potential impact you could have as a CMA in halting the spread of infectious diseases.

Biological Agents

When an infectious disease spreads, germs that may travel from one person to another or from animals to humans are responsible for spreading it. The following are the major organisms:

Viruses

Among the most prevalent infectious agents are viruses. They are tiny, harmful organisms that can harm bacteria, fungi, humans, animals, and birds. Although viruses are not living beings, they exhibit living characteristics. They were initially believed to be alive creatures, but scientists later discovered that they are actually sophisticated creatures that lay somewhere between living and non-living entities. The majority of viruses are made up of several components, mostly proteins and nuclei. When viruses attack, they can cause significant damage and are frequently challenging to treat.

Typically, a virus is composed of DNA and RNA and is encased in lipids, proteins, or glycoproteins. They are parasitic in nature and disease carriers. This explains why, once within the host's body, they constantly flourish.

One of the most prevalent biological species in the world is the virus. Most of the diseases they spread are incurable but treatable. There are numerous ways for viruses to spread from one person to another. The following are some examples of typical transmission methods:

Saliva interchange, physical contact with an infected person, the sharing of foods and drinks, sexual intimacy, and the transmission of diseases from one species of animal to another.

But how each virus spreads from one person to the next varies. For instance, greetings or sharing a dish cannot spread the Human Immunodeficiency Virus. Likewise, aerosol transmission is a way for the coronavirus that causes COVID-19 to spread from one person to another. Some viruses, such as the extremely contagious ebolavirus, require immediate management measures. Others, such as influenza, require long-term management plans to prevent them from spreading from one person to another.

Parasites

One of the typical infection-transmitting agents is the parasite. They are living things whose survival is entirely dependent on other living things. Alternatively put, parasites will reside within or above another living thing. It is typical for a parasite to switch between hosts. The parasites operate as agents of infection transfer by transferring infections from host A to host B as they travel around.

In addition to physically traveling from one host to another, parasites can also enter a host's body through food and drink. Some parasites can be acquired by consuming tainted food and drink, while others can be breathed in or picked up through skin contact. The majority of parasites are tiny in size, while others are very large and visible to the naked eye. The majority of parasites thrive and reach their full capacity inside the bodies of their hosts. Protozoa, hookworms, tapeworms, crabs, lice, and skin mites are a few examples of parasites.

Since parasites live and grow inside their hosts, they also weaken the hosts by putting an extra burden on them with worms and denying them of nutrition.

One of the main sources of infection transmission is bacteria. A bacteria is essentially a microscopic, live, disease-causing creature. Touch, saliva exchange, sexual contact, food, and water are all ways that bacteria can spread from one host to another. There are various kinds of bacteria that transmit various infections. The most prevalent bacterially transmitted illnesses include cholera, typhoid, gonorrhea, pneumonia, TB, and syphilis.

Although they are relatively common, bacterial infections are far simpler to treat than most viral infections. Antibiotics come in a variety of forms and are used to treat bacterial illnesses. While people use antibiotics regularly, it is important that the drug be prescribed by a doctor after ascertaining the exact condition that a patient is suffering from.

Fungi

Fungi are living organisms that can grow literally anywhere, including on land, on surfaces such as tables, on human skin, and inside the human body. Fungi are disease-carrying agents and can be quite dangerous when they attack the human body. Examples of fungi that can attack the human body include Aspergillus, candida, yeast, and mold.

One of the most prevalent fungi that affects the human body is dimorphic yeast. It can exist as either yeast or mold, depending on the environment. Among the fungal conditions that are common in the USA include Histoplasma, candida, and sporothrix. Others include athlete's foot and ringworms.

Fungi can be transferred from one person to another through physical contact or sexual intimacy. If you come in contact with a person who has ringworms, you may also get infected with the same organism.

Modes of Infection Transmission

There are various ways in which the agents of infections can be transferred from one person to another. The modes of infection transmission are:

Indirect Contact

Indirect contact simply means that the disease-transmitting agents can be passed from one person to another through interaction. In this mode of transmission, there does not necessarily need to be physical contact between the two parties. With indirect contact, a virus or bacteria can be passed just by being in the same environment. For instance, the organism could be transferred from a door handle that has been touched by an infected person, from the toilet seat, or from sharing personal care items.

Droplet Spread

Droplet spread is one of the most common ways of spreading infectious agents. When a person speaks, sneezes, or coughs, microscopic droplets may emanate from their mouth. If you are in close contact with this person, these droplets may land on your body or even in your mouth. Once inhaled, these airborne droplets may cause a lung infection.

This mode of transmission is very common in airborne diseases such as the common flu and coronavirus. As a result, airborne infections can quickly spread in the community.

Besides breath-based droplets, if an infected person leaves droplets of blood, saliva, or water on a surface, another person could get infected from it. This is the reason why high standards of sanitization for surfaces in health facilities are a must.

Person-to-Person Contact

Under indirect contact, there is also a possibility of person-to-person contact. This simply means that you may get into physical contact with a person even without knowledge. If you happen to hug a person who has an infectious agent on their body, there is a chance that the agent will be transferred to you. The same can happen when you come into contact with people with a fungal infection, lice, or scabies. These circumstances can lead to the spread of bacteria, viruses, bacteria, and fungi without your primary knowledge.

Direct Contact

Diseases that are transmitted through direct contact are referred to as contagious diseases. These are conditions that primarily thrive when the infected person comes in personal contact with other people. Further, the infectious agent can be transmitted through sharing of personal items. Among the personal effects that commonly transmit infections include sharing clothes, socks, towels, bathing rugs, razors, and combs.

Inhalation

Inhalation is one of the most common modes of transmitting infectious agents. The problem with inhalation is that it is much harder to control than is the case with the other modes of transmission. In this mode of infectious agent transmission, the only way to stop the agents from being transmitted to an individual is by staying away from infected individuals and wearing masks.

Under inhalation, infectious agents are passed from one person to another through coughing, sneezing, and talking. If a person coughs or sneezes in the air you are breathing; you are likely to inhale infected droplets from their mouth.

Vector-Borne Transmission

Lastly, another mode of transmitting infectious agents is via vectors. In this method, the bacteria, virus, fungi, or parasite carrying the disease is passed from one person to another through the help of wild and domestic animals or insects. When humans interact with animals, there are chances that they may acquire an infection. Common vector-borne disorders include Lyme disease, malaria, Rocky Mountain spotted fever, zika virus, and dengue.

Vector-borne diseases are among the leading causes of death in the world. They thrive in tropical and subtropical regions where there is warm weather and plenty of rain.

Ingestion is a mode of transmission of infectious agents in which a person swallows the disease-causing agents. This can happen through eating contaminated foods or drinking contaminated water. Foods and water may be contaminated by feces, saliva, or other bodily waste products and can easily lead to an infection. Classic examples include hepatitis A, amebiasis, traveler's diarrhea, bacterial food poisoning, and cholera.

Chain of Infection and Infection Control

Infectious agents generally can't survive outside the host for long periods. Even so, there is a chain that is followed for infections. There are six main links in the chain of infections. These links are:

Pathogen

A pathogen is a bacterium, virus, or any agent that can cause disease. This is the starting point in the link of infections.

Reservoir

The reservoir refers to an environment where the pathogen can survive. There are many places where a pathogen can survive. Among the places where pathogens can survive include the body of an animal, food, water bodies, contaminated soil/water, and bodies of humans. Among the most common animal reservoirs include cows, sheep, rabbits, dogs, and other domestic animals. They transmit several conditions, including anthrax, monkeypox, tularemia, and others.

Portal of Exit

There are various portals of exit on the human body. The portal of exit is determined by the type of pathogen in question. For instance, pathogens that affect the respiratory system exit through the mouth and the nose.

Means of Transmission

The means of transmission refers to the way through which the pathogen is transferred from the reservoir to the new host. In most cases, the pathogens may be acquired via contaminated food or water, inhalation, direct contact, sexual activity, etc.

Portal of Entry

The portal of entry is the point through which a pathogen enters its host. There are many portals of entry for humans. There are pathogens that can enter through the skin, like some fungi and parasites. There are other pathogens that can enter through the eyes, mouth, or reproductive organs. For most sexually transmitted infections, the reproductive organs are the point of entry. On the other hand, infections that are related to the respiratory system are mostly associated with the mouth and nose as points of entry.

New Host

The new host refers to the final destination where the pathogen settles. In this case, the final destination is the human body. The ability of pathogens to settle in the human body depends on various factors. Among the key factors of consideration are the genetics of the potential host and their overall body immunity. Individuals with a weak immune system are highly susceptible to pathogen attacks. In most cases, individuals who have a strong immune system may get attacked by pathogens but will not suffer from the disease or develop severe symptoms.

Infection Control

Since infections can be quite costly to manage in the long run, it is important to control their spread. Infection control is the process through which the spread and transmission of infectious agents are stopped or reduced. There are many approaches to infection control. In this section, we will just look at the key steps that CMAs can take to assist in infection control. Some of the ways in which infections are controlled include:

Maintain Hygiene

Simple hygiene measures go a long way in controlling infections. Among the ways of ensuring good hygiene include regular cleaning of personal effects such as bedsheets, clothing, and others. Secondly, ensure that your body is always cleaned especially after coming in contact with infected people. Given that most pathogens are transferred from people to other people, you can minimize the rate of transmission by always washing your hands after interacting with people.

There is also general cleanliness that must be observed in public spaces. In such facilities, general areas must be cleaned and disinfected regularly. These steps go a long way in ensuring that the surfaces touched by infected patients do not become conduits for transferring the same infections to other people.

Use Appropriate Personal Protective Equipment

Personal protective effects are very important for those who work in health facilities. In health facilities, the chances of getting infected are very high. As a CMA, you will meet all types of people suffering from various infectious disorders. The only sure way of remaining safe in your line of duty is by wearing personal protective gear.

There are several types of items that make up personal protective gear, including a pair of gloves, closed shoes, medical gowns, and facemasks. This protective wear can be quite important in reducing the chances of contact between you and your patients.

Waste Disposal

Finally, proper disposal of waste matter and contaminated syringes and needles is important in infection control. Waste disposal must be done in accordance with the best practices. In terms of medical waste, it is required that all types of waste are disposed of separately from other types of waste. You cannot dispose of medical waste in the same manner as the other types of waste found in homes. Further, medical wastewater should be sterilized before it is disposed of. Waste such as syringes and others must be sterilized before being released into the environment. Other wastes from medical facilities undergo treatment to ensure that there are no harmful pathogens moving outside the medical facility into the free world.

Summary

- Infection control is essential for various reasons, including reducing financial burdens, preventing deaths, and decreasing the strain on medical facilities.
- Infection control methods include isolation, mass vaccination, public health education, personal hygiene, and governmental regulations.
- Personal protective equipment (PPE) like gloves, gowns, and masks is crucial for healthcare workers to reduce the risk of infection transmission.
- Proper waste disposal, including sterilizing medical waste, is essential for infection control.
- Infections can be transmitted through indirect contact (surfaces), droplet spread (airborne), person-to-person contact, direct contact (contagious diseases), inhalation (airborne patho-

gens), vector-borne transmission (through animals or insects), and ingestion (contaminated food or water).

- The chain of infection consists of six links: pathogen, reservoir, portal of exit, means of transmission, portal of entry, and new host.
- Pathogens are disease-causing agents, and they can survive in various reservoirs, including animals and the environment.
- The means of transmission include contaminated food, water, inhalation, direct contact, sexual activity, etc.
- The portal of entry is where the pathogen enters the host, and the new host is where the pathogen settles.
- Host immunity plays a role in whether infection occurs or how severe it becomes.
- CMAs should maintain personal hygiene, wash hands regularly, and keep personal effects clean.
- The use of appropriate personal protective equipment (PPE) is crucial for CMAs working in healthcare settings.
- Proper waste disposal and sterilization of medical waste are essential components of infection control in healthcare facilities.
- These takeaways cover the fundamental aspects of infection control and understanding the spread of infectious agents, which are important topics for the CMA exam.

CHAPTER 11

Nutrition And Dietetics

A CRUCIAL COMPONENT of medical care is nutrition. A healthy diet should be suggested to patients by healthcare professionals. In this regard, it is expected of health professionals to have a fundamental knowledge of the nutritional needs of their patients.

Although nutritional specialists are not expected of CMAs, your exam will test your fundamental understanding of nutrition. The nutritional meals, supplements, and other dietary products that can benefit your patients are expected of you as a CMA.

Let's start by considering the value of nutrition before moving on to the sorts of food nutrients that are available and where they can be found.

Vitality of Nutrition

1. Promotes Longevity: Eating healthily raises one's general immunity. As a result, following a healthy diet increases the likelihood that a person will be able to fight off viruses that attack the body. Your body will be equipped to battle diseases if you eat the correct meals.
2. Maintains the Health of the Skin, Teeth, and Eyes: Each organ in your body requires particular nutrients to stay in good health. For instance, to nourish your skin, you must consume meals high in vitamin C. Likewise, calcium-rich diets will significantly strengthen your teeth. You should eat meals that support the organs in your body that require that support depending on your aim.
3. Supports Muscles: Your entire body mass is affected by the foods you consume. Distinct food varieties have distinct effects on the body. If you want to lose weight, you can eat some meals to activate weight reduction. Nutrition can also explain how much weight you gain.
4. Boosts Immunity: One of the most significant functions of diet is the control of an individual's immunity. Simply put, immunity is the body's capacity to fend off illnesses. You have low immunity if your body is very vulnerable to illness. There are foods, such as fruits, vitamins, minerals, etc., that help strengthen immunity.

5. Strengthening Bones: As a CMA, you can come across patients who have health issues that weaken their bones. Patients should be advised to eat meals high in calcium and vitamin D when treating such a condition.

6. Reduces Risk of Heart Disease: Poor diet may contribute to the development of diseases like heart disease, type 2 diabetes, and different forms of cancer. A Mediterranean diet is advised to reduce the risk of heart disease; this diet promotes fruits, vegetables, nuts, grains, and the usage of unsaturated fats; fish is favored over red meat.

7. Encourages Healthy Pregnancy: Those who provide care for expectant and lactating moms place a high value on nutrition and dietetics. The diet of a pregnant woman directly affects the health of the unborn child. It is advised to have a healthy, balanced diet when pregnant, with a focus on taking folate supplements to reduce the chance of the fetus developing neural tube abnormalities.

8. Aids in Digestive System Function: Getting the right diet is essential for a healthy digestive system. Constipation sufferers are advised to eat a diet rich in fiber. Dairy products should be avoided by individuals who are lactose intolerant while gluten-containing meals by those who have celiac disease.

Food Nutrients

There are six basic categories used to group all human meals. Based on the food's nutritional value, a classification is made. Specific nutrients are offered by each type of food. CMAs are expected to have a solid understanding of the foods that are readily available, their advantages for health, and their complete nutritional profiles. Here are the six groups of foods according to their nutritional value.

Carbohydrates

Foods high in carbohydrates give the body instant energy. These foods contain carbon, hydrogen, and oxygen in their molecules. Foods that fall under the category of carbs are numerous.

- Starches: Foods that contain starches are those that contain long-chain glucose molecules. Humans' digestive systems convert them into glucose when they ingest them.

- Sugars: Sugars are short-chain carbohydrates that are crucial for the overall energy and sugar balance of your body. Fructose, sucrose, and glucose are some examples of sugars.

- Fiber: The digestive system of a human is not designed to process fiber. However, some of the bacteria in our gut have a variety of uses for fiber. Vegetables and some grains contain fibers.

In addition to being foods that are high in energy, carbohydrates are also some of the most widely available foods. Foods like rice, cereals, nuts, fruits, vegetables, and grains are examples of common carbs.

In light of this, it's crucial to understand that there are healthy and unhealthy carbohydrates. Some sources of carbs include fruits, vegetables, nuts, fiber, and whole grains. If you're going to consume them, look for healthy carbs. Those selections with too much sugar are harmful or those with bad carbs. White bread, pastries, ice cream, sweet beverages, and other foods high in sugar are examples of these carbs. Foods high in processed sugars are generally bad for your health. To ensure that your patients benefit the most from your therapies, you should be able to advise them on the best carbs as a CMA.

Proteins

Proteins make up the second category of the foods we eat. The nutrients that compose the structural components of our bodies are proteins. They support the growth of bones, cells, hair, and muscles. Your daily diet should be largely composed of proteins, but they shouldn't ever be the only item on the table.

Sixteen percent (16%) of the weight of the human body is made up of proteins. The human body needs these proteins for growth and development. Protein is essential for growing and developing healthily, and it aids in the healing of wounds. There are several distinct types of proteins in the human body. These proteins all have various functions.

Protein-rich foods are widely available and can assist in fueling our bodies. Some grains can also be good sources of protein, in addition to meat-based diets. For the human body, soy, beans, certain grains, nuts, and meat-based items are the primary sources of protein. There are healthy proteins and unhealthy proteins, just like there are both. The proteins in grains like soy and beans are good proteins. Some forms of meat, especially red meat, contain bad proteins.

In its simplest form, the term "protein" merely denotes a mixture of amino acids. The human body does not keep amino acids despite the fact that it needs them. By altering the available amino acids, it creates them. It is crucial to ingest proteins for this reason. Humans use foods high in protein to obtain nine essential amino acids. These amino acids include histidine, tryptophan, methionine, lysine, valine, threonine, isoleucine, and leucine.

A healthy adult needs 0.8 grams of protein for every kilogram of body weight. For example, a person weighing 30 kg needs (0.8 x 30) grams of protein each day.

Fats

The third category of healthy foods includes fats. Fats were first considered to be harmful to the body. Recent research, however, has demonstrated the value of fats in a balanced diet. All people are advised to eat certain healthy fats.

Adults should not include more than 30% of fat in their diet, per the World Health Organization. Furthermore, it matters what kind of fats are being discussed. Like with proteins and carbohydrates, there are good and bad fats. Good carbohydrates aid in controlling blood sugar, which subsequently helps to ward off type 2 diabetes.

The use of healthy fats has many advantages. In addition to reducing the risk of diabetes, fats provide the body with energy. Additionally, they aid in lowering the risk of a variety of illnesses like certain malignancies, Alzheimer's disease, and arthritis. The following are many categories of fats:

Saturated fats

High hydrogen atom concentrations are a characteristic of saturated lipids. Plants like coconuts, meat-based foods like beef and chicken, processed meats like hot dogs, dairy products like cheese and butter, and some pre-packaged snacks are the main sources of saturated fats.

Depending on the kind of fats consumed, saturated fats might hurt a person's health. For instance, consuming dairy fats lowers the risk of developing cardiovascular illnesses. In addition, consuming processed meats like sausage and bacon increases the chance of developing cardiovascular disorders.

Unsaturated fats

Compared to saturated fats, unsaturated fats contain fewer hydrogen atoms. In contrast to saturated fats, which continue to exist in a solid form at room temperature, they are often liquid. Additionally, they are divided into monounsaturated and polyunsaturated fats. While monounsaturated fats only have one bond, polyunsaturated fats have two.

Monounsaturated fats are found in foods including olive oil, canola oil, avocados, various types of seeds, and nuts. The oils from corn and sunflower are examples of polyunsaturated fats.

Vitamins

The human body requires vitamins for proper development. Different forms of food contain vitamins, which are necessary for growth. There are 13 vitamins in the human body, including vitamins A, B, C, D, E, and K. While the body produces some of these vitamins, the majority are obtained from the foods we eat.

It's critical to keep an eye on your vitamin consumption because failing to do so can result in a vitamin shortage. For instance, a lack of vitamin C might have an impact on your skin and make it more prone to damage. The following are the categories for vitamins:

Fat-soluble vitamins

Those vitamins that can dissolve in fat are said to be fat-soluble. The liver and other fatty tissues of the body contain these vitamins, which are often dissolved in body fat. They can be stored for a few months.

Water-soluble vitamins

The opposite of fat-soluble vitamins is a water-soluble vitamin. Only water is capable of dissolving these vitamins. They can't stay in the body for very long as a result, and the liver or kidneys swiftly eliminate them. They should be constantly refilled because they are readily eliminated. This is why a person should consume a specified range of vitamin-rich meals on a regular basis.

Vitamins C, B$_1$, B$_1$, B$_1$, B$_2$, B$_6$, B$_2$, B$_9$, and B$_3$ are the essential water-soluble vitamins that the human body needs. Whole grains, brown rice, oranges, spinach, broccoli, and sunflower seeds are among the excellent sources of these vitamins. Beriberi, scurvy, and rickets are a few of the illnesses that might strike a person who does not consume enough vitamins.

Minerals

Minerals are the body's fourth nutritional supplement category. Minerals are used by our bodies for a variety of functions, including metabolism. Minerals are needed to keep the health of the muscles, bones, brain, heart, and other body systems. The majority of the body's organs depend on minerals to perform vital tasks including the synthesis of enzymes. Trace minerals and macro-minerals are additional categories for minerals.

Trace minerals

The body needs trace minerals in tiny amounts. Iron, cobalt, selenium, fluoride, zinc, iodine, and other trace minerals are necessary. Food and water are the main sources of trace minerals.

Macro-minerals

Magnesium, sodium, potassium, calcium chloride, and phosphorus are examples of macro-minerals that the body requires in rather high amounts. They play a number of functions, including maintaining physiological fluids, constructing strong bones, and turning food into energy.

Water

The sixth and last division of dietary requirements is water. Although water is not a food, it is vital to the body's health. Numerous crucial functions that water fulfills in the human body include:

- Transportation: Nutrients are transported throughout the body via water. Because they are water-soluble, the majority of nutrients are eaten in water and absorbed in the blood.

- Detoxification: The body uses water for this vital additional function. You can use your urine to flush away more toxins if you drink enough water each day. Simply put, constant urination refers to the body's removal of extra toxins.

- Lubrication: Water is the sole substance that can serve as a consistent source of lubrication for the majority of bodily organs. Our eyes, mouths, lips, sex organs, and joints are all lubricated by water. Organs like the liver and lungs cannot function if they become dehydrated.

- Avert Dehydration: The absence of enough water in the body is referred to as dehydration. You can prevent the body from being dehydrated by drinking lots of water. Low blood pressure, sluggishness, headaches, blurred vision, and muscle weakness are all symptoms of dehydration.

- Prevents Constipation: Undigested and digested meals might cause constipation when they enter your colon. Dehydration is one of the main causes of constipation.

- It is advised that eight glasses of water each day are taken by adults.

Special Dietary Needs

Dietary requirements for those with particular medical disorders are referred to as special dietary needs. Some folks can't survive on a typical diet. To thrive, some people need particular diets. For instance, a person with celiac disease must adhere to a gluten-free diet at all times. CMAs are essential in making sure that patients' dietary requirements are addressed.

Weight Control Diet

People frequently embark on diets to lose weight. Most of the time, when we talk about weight control, the goal is to lose weight by dietary adjustments. Patients who are trying to control their weight may benefit from eating some of the following foods:

- Vegetables such as kale, spinach, broccoli, and Swiss chard are the majority of leafy greens. Although they are largely low-calorie, these foods are also nutrient-dense. Greens are strongly advised for anyone who is having weight problems. Additionally, you ought to make an effort to limit your intake of carbs. Greens have the advantage of being low in carbohydrates while still being fulfilling. Because they have high fiber content, they can keep a person satisfied for a long time. In addition to all of these crucial details, most greens also include minerals and antioxidants. Antioxidants aid in fat metabolism and aid the body in shedding extra fat that contributes to obesity.

- Beans and other legumes are advised for maintaining a healthy weight. The key justification is that they provide a good substitution for conventional sources of protein. Despite being high in protein, beans and other legumes are healthier than animal alternatives. The majority of meat-based protein sources are unhealthy for the body and are likely to make people gain too much weight. Additionally, beans and other legumes are high in fiber and provide the consumer with a prolonged feeling of satiety. The constant want to eat is one of the main problems that weight control attempts to solve. Utilizing legumes like beans is one method to reduce the daily amount of food you consume. Soy, French beans, and kidney beans are a few of the items you can eat.

- The greatest grain substitute for refined grains is whole grain. For those who want to lose weight, they are the best source of carbohydrates. Whole grains are wonderful because they have high fiber content. The fiber eases constipation, decreases the desire to eat, and increases satiety. Additionally, the fiber in these foods speeds up the body's digestion of food. You can consume basic whole-grain items like oats, brown rice, and brown bread.

- Fruits are a healthy meal option for body nutrition and weight management. Some fruits have very high natural sugar content. Natural sugar, however, is far healthier for the body than processed sugar. While some fruits may naturally contain sugar, all fruits include fiber, which regulates the body's absorption of sugar. Additionally, the fiber makes sure that you stay fuller for extended periods of time, which lowers the rate of food consumption.

Hypertension

Plaque accumulation in the arteries results in hypertension, also referred to as high blood pressure. Consuming foods high in cholesterol contributes to the accumulation of fat. A family history and a lack of exercise are further contributing factors. When a person has hypertension, certain meals must be avoided and only healthy options should be consumed. High blood pressure can cause a stroke if preventative measures like diet control are not performed. This is the justification for requesting that all patients with this ailment eat low-cholesterol diets. The following foods are among those advised for those with high blood pressure:

- Fruits are highly recommended for those with hypertension. This is a result of their low carb, high fiber, and low cholesterol content. Doctors advise consuming fruits unprocessed and in their natural state. Such organic fruits are the greatest because they decrease your propensity to overeat.

- Whole grains are excellent for those with high blood pressure. Due to their high fiber content, whole grains should not be consumed in large quantities. The fiber can prolong your feeling of being fuller, which decreases your desire to constantly eat. In addition to having fiber, essential nutrients can also be sourced from whole grains.

- Nuts are a fantastic supply of fats that don't put your life in danger from high blood pressure. The beauty of nuts is how gratifying they are. Additionally, nuts are a natural source of a few minerals and omega fatty acids that the body needs to maintain blood circulation.

- Chicken and fish High blood pressure sufferers can consume some proteins, but not all of them. White meat, which has less fat than red meat, is the best option for them to eat. The suggested meat choices are fish and chicken. These people are also free to consume poultry products like eggs. However, the majority of these poultry products need to be cooked thoroughly.

- Low-fat goods: Most importantly, stay away from high-fat foods if you have high blood pressure. Avoid high-fat foods, such as any sort of meat that is fatty, and limit your use of butter. If you must eat fats, stick to unsaturated fats (the healthiest type). Additionally, all of your meals should be prepared with unsaturated fats like olive oil, which is liquid at room temperature.

People with hypertension should absolutely avoid some foods. Patients with high blood pressure should specifically avoid high-fat diets. Other foods that hypertensive people should avoid include the following:

- Simple Sugars: If you have high blood pressure, stay away from any foods that have sugar added to them. In essence, this will comprise the vast majority of pastries, soft drinks, and even certain alcoholic beverages. If any of the items you eat at home have added sugars, your blood pressure can increase.

- Red Meat: If you have high blood pressure, you must also stay away from red meat. The majority of red meat contains "bad cholesterol," which can readily accumulate in your blood vessels and cause blockage. Blood channel blockages cause high blood pressure. While some meat can be consumed by hypertension individuals, red meat consumption should be restricted. If you must eat meat, limit your food consumption to white meats like fowl or fish.

- Sweets and foods high in sugar: Finally, those with hypertension should avoid high-sugar foods. Avoid any sweets and foods with added sugars in particular. Even if you have hypertension, there are some fruits you can eat. The majority of highly sugared fruits must be avoided, nevertheless. Apples, watermelons, plums, and prunes are a few of the fruits that doctors advise hypertension patients to consume.

Cancer

Cancers come in different forms, and they typically result in appetite reduction and weight loss. Cancer patients have special dietary requirements since they lose a lot of weight while also losing their appetite. In order to hasten the healing process, food is required. The mass wasting caused by cancer therapies like chemotherapy must also be considered. Patients must therefore consume foods that aid in regaining their lost mass. The following foods are among those advised for cancer patients:

- Vegetables: Greens and leaves are crucial for cancer sufferers. They want vitamin-rich foods that can significantly assist them in rejuvenating biological functioning when they shed a significant amount of weight. Greens are essential for supporting regular processes even if they do not help regenerate deteriorated tissue. Without minerals, the body's blood flow is impeded and its ability to perform its activities is also limited.

- Protein-rich meals are likely the most crucial for cancer patients. Proteins are essential for cancer patients in order to rebuild damaged tissues. The drug therapy eliminates not only cancer cells but also healthy cells, which may have a number of unfavorable effects, such as hair loss and weight loss. Proteins are essential for helping cancer patients rebuild their muscle mass. Proteins are essential for regaining their full stature.
White meat alternatives like fish, beans, and soy, dairy items like yogurt and cheese, and poultry products like chicken and eggs are among the high-protein foods advised for cancer patients. If a cancer patient also has another ailment, it should be considered when

making suggestions. Dairy products are advised for cancer patients; however, they might not be the best choice for those who have high blood pressure. Therefore, speaking with a dietitian is crucial.

- Plenty of Water: Patients with cancer also need to eat and drink regularly. Cancer patients who don't eat right typically fare poorly, not because of their illness but rather because they don't have enough energy to keep their bodies running. Patients who do not drink enough water risk dehydration, anuria, lethargy, and hypotension. Additionally, water aids in the body's detoxification process.

Lactose-Intolerant Individuals

A form of sugar called lactose is frequently present in dairy milk. Some people struggle to easily digest this sugar. By lactase enzymes, this sugar must be broken down in the digestive tract. Foods high in lactose may cause issues for people who don't have enough lactase enzymes. They frequently have issues with bloating, vomiting, diarrhea, and stomach pains. These symptoms can be rather unpleasant, which is why some people are thought to be lactose intolerant.

Milk and other dairy products like cheese and butter are at the top of the list of foods to stay away from. Other foods, including dairy products, also have high lactose content. These consist of sauces, beer, sweeteners, gravy, and canned tuna.

The market offers a wide variety of lactose-free meals. The majority of lactose-free goods may be made from cow's milk. Ask a store about them or hunt for a speciality store if you're looking for foods that are perfect for lactose intolerant people. Even milk and cheese that has undergone thorough processing to accommodate lactose intolerant people is available.

Eating Disorders

People with eating problems may follow specific food regimens. While medical professionals are free to suggest appropriate diets for eating disorder patients, the majority of these people also have a variety of mental issues that need to be treated. The patient must attend therapy sessions to address the underlying psychological issue in order to treat an eating disorder. These disorders are typically brought on by an odd fascination with one's physique. Eating disorders come in six different primary categories. They consist of the following:

- Anorexia Nervosa: Anorexia Nervosa is an eating condition that primarily affects females. People who have this illness often avoid particular foods and see themselves as being overweight. Malnutrition frequently comes from this.
- Binge Eating: Binge eating is a mental health issue that affects children and teenagers. It alludes to consuming a lot of food all at once.
- Rumination Disorder: A person with this sort of disorder exhibits ruminant behavior. In essence, they consume and swallow the food they have just regurgitated. This can happen at any point in life.
- Bulimia Nervosa: Another eating disorder that is extremely similar to binge disorder is bulimia nervosa. But this particular eating disorder differs from others in that its victims do not lose weight. Instead, they keep their weight rather constant throughout.
- Pica: Patients with this eating problem, known as pica, often have cravings for items other than food. People who have this illness frequently consume soil, paper, pens, and other items.
- Avoidant Disorder: A patient with an avoidant disorder, sometimes referred to as a restrictive disorder, refrains from eating because they don't like specific tastes or colors. People who have this illness might not eat because they don't like particular colors.

Summary

- A healthy diet promotes longevity and boosts overall immunity.
- Specific nutrients are essential for the health of various organs, such as vitamin C for the skin and calcium for teeth.
- Nutrition influences body weight and can be tailored to achieve weight loss or weight gain.
- A well-balanced diet supports a strong immune system and disease resistance.
- Adequate calcium and vitamin D intake is vital for bone health.
- Following a Mediterranean diet can assist in the reduction of the risk of heart disease.
- Proper nutrition is required during pregnancy to support the development of the fetus.
- Dietary choices play a vital role in maintaining a healthy digestive system.

- Carbohydrates provide immediate energy and can be found in foods like rice, cereals, fruits, and vegetables.
- Proteins are essential for growth, muscle development, and wound healing; sources include soy, beans, nuts, and certain meats.
- Fats are necessary in moderation, with good fats like unsaturated fats being beneficial for health.
- Vitamins are essential for various bodily functions and can be fat-soluble or water-soluble.
- Minerals, including trace minerals and macro-minerals, are crucial for metabolism and organ function.
- Water is vital for nutrient transportation, detoxification, and overall bodily function.
- Weight control diets should emphasize greens, beans, whole grains, and fruits to manage weight effectively.
- Hypertension patients should consume low-cholesterol, high-fiber, and low-sugar foods while avoiding high-fat and sugary items.
- Cancer patients require nutrient-rich foods, especially greens, protein sources like white meat and dairy, and adequate hydration.
- Lactose-intolerant individuals should avoid dairy products and opt for lactose-free alternatives.
- Eating disorders come in various forms. Each of them requires a specific dietary and psychological approach for treatment.

CHAPTER 12

Pharmacology Part 2

THE STUDY OF drugs and the various effects they have on their users is known as pharmacology. The study of pharmacology requires more time than a few days due to its breadth. CMAs aren't required to be pharmacologists, though. On the other hand, they are simply required to have a basic understanding of the medicines that are accessible and how using them affects persons who use them.

What Exactly Is Pharmacology?

Pharmacology encompasses several academic fields that are all concerned with medicines and how they work to treat patients. As a CMA, you should base your knowledge of pharmacology on the following three points:

Drug Class Categories

This simply implies that you should be able to categorize different drugs as necessary. It is simpler to work if you group medications into broad classes. You will be able to identify which medications fall under which group and comprehend how they are administered thanks to classification. Even though this information is relatively basic, it can be highly important in situations where a doctor is not available.

Drug Retention

As a CMA, you must next consider medicine storage. As we will see momentarily, each drug class has unique storage needs. The medications could readily spoil if the maintenance and storage standards are not satisfied. Patients may experience harm from tainted medications. You will be tested on your understanding of medication storage as a CMA. Additionally, information on how the majority of medication classes are handled and kept must be provided.

Drug Reactions

You must, above all else, be familiar with the many kinds of drug reactions. Drug responses are largely influenced by the patient's gender, age, and other characteristics. CMAs are expected to have a general awareness of how particular drug classes are likely to interact with a particular population of patients.

Classes of Drugs

Patients' medications are often divided into six classes. Your work as a CMA will be relatively simple if you comprehend these classifications and what they stand for. The following are the drug classes:

Antidepressants

There are various depressants, and they range in potency. In essence, these medications function by preventing the breakdown of specific neurotransmitters. The person feels happier when this occurs.

One of the most commonly used medications all over the world is a depressant. Tricyclic antidepressants, SSRIs (Selective Serotonin reuptake inhibitors), atypical antidepressants, monoamine oxidase inhibitors, and SNRIs (serotonin and norepinephrine reuptake inhibitors) are some of the common antidepressants.

Barbiturates

These medicines inhibit the central nervous system. Their primary responsibility is to induce sleep and relaxation in a patient. Today, barbiturates are rarely utilized due to their poor safety profile. These substances can also result in physical dependence. Since they are regarded as prohibited substances, doctors rarely prescribe them.

Worldwide, the most commonly used psychoactive substance is ethanol, or alcohol as it is more commonly known. A psychoactive chemical called ethyl alcohol has the potential to damage one's capacity for judgment. Although it is frequently used at large doses as a disinfectant, this medication is not utilized medically. Alcohol is typically consumed for leisure. The fact that alcohol is addictive poses the most risk. Those who drink should exercise caution to avoid developing an addiction to it.

Benzodiazepines

These are a class of psychoactive medications used in medicine to treat conditions like stress, sleeplessness, anxiety, and muscular spasms. A condition called insomnia causes people to lose sleep. Insomniacs frequently struggle with underlying mental and emotional problems. One of the few approaches to putting a patient to sleep is to employ such psychotropic medications.

The most popular sedatives in the US are benzodiazepines. They also benefit patients who are stressed out or anxious. Users of these medicines experience both immediate and long-term effects. Fatigue, depression, fever, reduced blood pressure, urinary issues, difficulty concentrating, sluggish motion, and addiction are a few of the side effects of drugs on users.

Depressants do have some positive effects while having so many undesirable side effects. The benefits of these medications are the main reasons people use them. Users are likely to enjoy the following benefits:

- Reduced anxiety
- Inhibited insomnia
- Inhibited seizures
- Controls social phobia
- Controls obsessive-compulsive disorder

These medications are perfect for anyone with any kind of mental or social impairment. Unfortunately, people who are not patients also use depressants. In contrast, due to these medications' sedative effects, many regular people abuse them. No patient should ever be prescribed a depressant without a doctor's approval. If you observe a patient taking drugs, you should be able to offer advice.

Stimulants

A class of medications known as stimulants can momentarily improve someone's energy and alertness. Stimulants are accessible with a prescription as tablets, capsules, and even injections. The patient's needs determine the sort of stimulant that is utilized. In light of this, most countries forbid the use of stimulants for recreation. The two stimulants that are most frequently abused are cocaine and amphetamines. Stimulants have certain negative side effects when misused. Increased alertness, increased heartbeat, decreased hunger, euphoria, and an excessive desire to converse are a few of these negative effects.

Paranoia is the most frequent adverse reaction to stimulant overdose. This can manifest in many ways, such as dread, delusions, and hallucinations. Higher stimulant doses can cause coma, convulsions, and anxiety. These medications have the potential to be fatal in the worst-case situation. Therefore, it's crucial to carefully control your stimulant intake. To prevent unintentional overdose, the medications should always be kept out of the reach of minors.

The most common side effect of overdosing on stimulants is paranoia. This can be shown in several ways, including hallucinations, delusions, and fear. Taking higher doses of stimulants can result in coma, seizures, and anxiety. In the worst-case scenario, these drugs can result in death. It is, therefore, important to monitor the intake of stimulants closely. The drugs should also be kept away from children at all times to avoid accidental overdose.

Inhalants

The term "inhalant" refers to any drug that may be inhaled and has the effect of modifying the user's state of consciousness. The blood often absorbs the chemical vapor that has been breathed. It moves through the entire body before affecting the nervous system. Inhalants provide certain advantages for the user, but they also have negative effects that can be fatal. They can result in lasting brain damage if not regulated. Several inhalants include:

Aerosols: In essence, these are substances that can be inhaled into the body from the outside world. Spray paint, hair sprays, deodorant sprays, cleaning supplies, and vegetable oils are some of them.

Solvents: Solvents are a component of items that can be ingested by inhalation and have an impact on a person's health and functioning. Gasoline, paint remover, dry cleaning fluids, lighter fluid, and paint thinner are some of the solvents that are frequently inhaled.

Another class of inhalants that is frequently employed for its psychedelic effects on users is nitrates. They consist of things like video head cleaners and room deodorizers.

Gases: The majority of the gases we breathe in have the power to affect how the body normally functions. Some gases are employed as inhalants specifically. They consist of whipped cream aerosols, butane lighters, ether, nitrous oxide, chloroform, and nitrous oxide. Inhalants have many side effects. The majority of inhalants have a direct impact on the central nervous system, which results in euphoria, lack of coordination, dizziness, and garbled speech.

There may be some long-term impacts of inhalants as well. Those who regularly inhale such chemicals run the danger of developing the following conditions: brain damage, kidney damage, hearing loss, liver damage, and delayed behavioral development in children.

Hallucinogens

These medications have a high likelihood of producing hallucinations. A person's emotions are known to fluctuate constantly when using hallucinogens. While some hallucinogens are artificial, others are found naturally. Many different kinds of mushrooms contain hallucinogens. They were traditionally employed in ceremonies and healing. People have recently turned to hallucinogens for educational objectives.

Several of the typical hallucinogens are:

- Mescaline: This is a chemical that is naturally present in the peyote cactus, a particular species of cactus. There is a disc-shaped area of the plant where mescaline is present in significant amounts. The disc is dried and submerged in water to extract the medication. The same medicine can be produced synthetically as well.
- Psilocybin: Psilocybin is a hallucinogen that can predominantly be found in certain types of mushrooms. The production of this chemical can also be done synthetically.

- LSD: D-lysergic acid diethylamide is one of the hallucinogens that is most frequently abused. It is a strong synthetic substance that is frequently overused; however, it has a lot of negative side effects. Daydreaming, hallucinations, anxiety, and other negative symptoms are a few of them.

Cannabis

Cannabis falls within the final drug group. They are sometimes known as marijuana and are among the most misused drugs in the world. Due to its lack of medical advantages and significant potential for misuse, this medicine is listed as a schedule 1 restricted substance. All organ systems in the body may be impacted by cannabis. More than 120 active chemicals in the medicine have the potential to impact how the body functions. Cannabidiol and THC are the cannabis compounds that have gone through the most extensive research. The plant's leaves and blooms are its most powerful components.

Cannabis appears to have some medical benefits, despite the fact that it has many negative effects on users. This explains why more nations have recently legalized marijuana. Cannabis can treat motion sickness, chronic pain, anxiety, and sleep difficulties. Legal cannabis use is only permitted to treat a specific type of seizure. Cannabis has been legalized in several states but not by the federal government for medical purposes.

Compared to therapeutic marijuana, recreational marijuana has a greater number of negative impacts on consumers.

Marijuana frequently has negative side effects, such as impaired cognitive function, underweight births, hallucinations, impaired body organs, and irrational decision-making.

To feel high is the primary motivation for recreational marijuana use. Users experience euphoria due to the THC in the plant.

Drug Storage Techniques

As vital as the drug itself is, drug storage is also crucial. The lack of pharmaceuticals is simply indicated by the proper medications being stored incorrectly. When dealing with various medications, it is important to keep in mind that they are stored in various conditions. CMAs are needed to possess a foundational understanding of drug storage in all contexts.

Understanding the variables that affect the stored medications is the first step in proper drug storage. Elements like temperature, moisture, and light influence how medications are stored.

No universal rule exists that can be used to store all medications. Contrarily, each type of medicine needs a certain set of environmental conditions when being stored. Comply with the manufacturer's instructions to be certain that you are using the proper amount of storage. On the box or directions page, the majority of medicine makers list the recommended storage conditions.

When discussing drug storage conditions, a few common words are employed. For instance, you might encounter instructions that say to store the product at room temperature or in a cool, dry environment. "Room temperature" falls in the range of 15 to 25 degrees Celsius in the pharmaceuticals should be kept in storage. The suggested temperatures range from 2 to 8 degrees Celsius if it says to store in a cool environment. The best storage temperature for refrigerated medications is between –10 and –25 degrees Celsius.

One of the most frequent instructions on medication packaging is to keep it out of children's reach and in a cool, dry environment. The only requirement for storing medications in a cool, dry environment is to keep them away from light. The components of medications could potentially deteriorate if they are not maintained properly. This specifically occurs when they are exposed to strong sunshine or high temperatures.

Proper medication storage has the following advantages:

Loss prevention: If medications are not stored properly, they might be lost in a variety of ways. Remember that the majority of medications are valuable and can be stolen. Make sure the expensive items are stored securely if you want to avoid theft. Damage may result in losses in addition to material loss. A significant loss of pharmaceuticals might result from water or fire damage.

Preserve medicine potency: All medications must always have the appropriate level of potency. Simply said, a drug's potency refers to how well all of its active ingredients continue to work. The medicine becomes less effective when the active ingredients weaken.

When kept in the proper conditions, medications keep their effectiveness. The following are the main environmental aspects to think about when keeping drugs:

- Lighting: The use of lighting is crucial for storing medications. The majority of medications should be kept out of direct sunlight but in areas with enough lighting. Drugs are typically kept in darker settings.
- Temperature: The next important aspect of the environment is temperature. Some medications must be kept in a cold storage facility under all circumstances. When handling such pharmaceuticals, make sure they are in their proper setting always. You must have a backup emergency plan in place if you reside in a region where power outages are frequent.
- Cleanliness: Environmental issues aside, all medications must be stored in a clean atmosphere. Failure to maintain a clean environment around the medicine could result in many issues. For instance, medications stored in a filthy, wet environment may develop mold.
- Humidity: Another crucial environmental condition to take into account while storing your medications is humidity. A location with a lot of moisture in the air is not good for growing pharmaceuticals. At the same time, extremely dry air is bad for storing medications. Drugs that need to stay hydrated may get dehydrated when the air is too dry. Drugs that should stay dry could become dampened when the air is excessively humid. If medications aren't being stored in a cool atmosphere, they should ideally be maintained in a cool, dry spot. Ensure that the location is dry if you are keeping them in a cold facility.

Drug Adverse Reactions

Adverse medication responses can occur from time to time. It is challenging to predict who will experience a negative drug reaction, and because various people react differently, the symptoms of a negative drug reaction might range from minor to severe. Therefore, careful monitoring is required when introducing a new medicine to a patient. The underlying (idiosyncratic) cause of a bad medication reaction is typically unknown. An allergic reaction is one of the most typical adverse drug reactions, underscoring the significance of asking every patient about their whole drug history.

Drug Reactions' Severity: Determining Factors

Drug effects might be mild or serious. Even after an overdose, some people's drug reactions may be mild, while others may experience significant side effects from even a very small quantity. The degree to which a person's body can metabolize substances is different for each person. The following elements affect a person's response to drugs:

1. Drug Factors: The drug itself is the primary determinant in determining how severe a drug reaction will be. For instance, how medications are administered matters. The type of medicine, the dosage, and the frequency of usage are further considerations. It is advised that patients purchase medications from legitimate pharmacies and carefully follow the usage directions to prevent drug-related problems. For instance, one should adhere to the doctor's recommended dosage of two tablets every day. Resuming the medication after skipping it for a day can create negative results.

2. Hereditary characteristics: Some characteristics are largely influenced by the patient's ancestry. Most medication allergies run in families. A person is more likely to get asthma if they are born into a family with asthmatic parents than if they do not. As a result, there is a substantial probability of an unfavorable drug reaction in someone who has a family history of allergies.

3. Illnesses: The state of one's health also affects how a medicine will behave. It's critical to ascertain whether the patient has hepatic or renal impairment before providing a certain medication. These people might not be able to excrete or break down the medication, causing large levels to build up and cause toxicity.

4. Patient Age: A patient's age influences how a person will respond to a drug. The liver, which has poor function in both the elderly and children, puts them at risk for negative medication reactions. For instance, the elderly person may not be able to break down the medication, or the infant's kidneys may not be fully developed.

5. Polypharmacy: There is a considerable chance of drug interactions that might result in toxicity and unfavorable reactions when patients are given numerous medications.

Physicians' Desk Reference (PDR)

A large book known as The Physician's Desk Reference is released every year to serve as a reference for doctors. It is a list of all medications that are legal in the US. The FDA has given its approval to every medicine in the book, which was published with the aid of pharmaceutical firms.

Every physician, including CMAs, has to read this vital book. The information includes specifics on some things, such as the following:

- The drug's manufacturer
- The drug's name
- The dosage requirements for the drug for people of all ages
- Pharmacokinetics
- Adverse reactions brought on by each drug
- The DEA class, which determines whether a drug can be used with a prescription or without
- Drug interactions
- The supply chain for the drugs
- Each state's contact information

When CMAs are unfamiliar with a medicine, they might utilize such literature as references.

For ease of usage, the PDR is segmented into sections. The following are the book's major divisions:

- Section 1: The first section contains information on the manufacturer, including their name, address, phone number, and other facts.
- Section 2: All of the drug pages in the book are listed here. This part is crucial since it serves as a reference for medications whose names you might not be familiar with. Find out more about them by looking them up on the information pages.
- Section 3: This section lists the many product categories in the book. Section three of the book contains information that can be found there if you know the name of a drug but are unsure of which category it falls under.

- Section 4: This is referred to as the section on product identification. The names of the manufacturers, the products' images, and other details can be used for medication identification. If you're curious about a specific substance but don't know what it looks like, just visit this area to learn more about it.

- Section 5: The fifth portion of the book is perhaps the most significant. You may find a summary of each drug's details in this section. The information includes, among other things, the drug's uses, dose, and age ranges that it is appropriate for. Drugs can also be distinguished from one another based on how they are categorized, used, and substituted.

- Section 6: The part must contain details about how the medication affects a patient after administration. Along with other things, it describes the procedures to be taken while doing drug administration.

Drug Administration

There are numerous approaches to administering drugs. The effectiveness of a medicine depends on how it is taken. The manner of administration depends on the kind of drugs in consideration as well. While some medications are taken orally, others may need to be injected. The patient's condition also affects how a medicine is delivered. Some people can take oral medications, while others might not be able to.

How to Give Medicines

The typical steps to administer medication are listed below:

- Orally administered: The most typical drug administration method is oral. The substances can be drunk, chewed, or ingested whole. Tablets and syrups are two examples of medications that are taken orally. For oral ingestion, liquids, pills, and even capsules work best. When a medicine is taken orally, it is digested as normal food. All medications enter the liver through the gut walls for absorption. The medications may undergo chemical breakdown in the liver (first pass effect) before being transported through the blood to the rest of the body.

- Subcutaneous Route: This is a technique for administering medication that involves injecting a liquid medicine under the skin. The medicine then travels to the rest of the body through the blood arteries. This type of administration is frequently utilized for people who are unable to swallow or for medications like insulin that may be broken down by the stomach.

- Intramuscular Injection: Another drug delivery technique that is best for administering big doses of medication is intramuscular injection. The medication is injected into the subcutaneous muscles. The thighs, upper arm muscles, or buttocks are typically the target locations when an intramuscular injection is utilized. When compared to injections under the skin, this approach is far more effective at allowing the drug to be absorbed. However, the blood flow in the areas where the injections were made is what determines how quickly the medicine is absorbed.

- Vaginal Route: Certain circumstances call for the administration of medication via the vagina. A tablet gel or ring is inserted into the vagina with this method of administration. This method is primarily employed to treat persistent vaginal infections such as yeast infections and UTIs. Other times, menopausal medications like estrogen are given using this technique. When administered intravaginally, these medications are significantly more effective and have fewer side effects than when taken orally.

- Intravenous(IV) Drug Administration: The most efficient way of administration is intravenous (IV) drug administration. In this method, the medication is injected right into the bloodstream. Intravenous injections have various advantages. This kind of injection initially improves accuracy. The blood circulation system receives the medication directly. Second, the mechanism guarantees that the medicine will act quickly. Contrary to intramuscular injection, which may take some time for the medicine to begin acting in the body, intravenous administration produces an immediate effect.

How to Select the Drug Administration Method

The best way to administer medication depends on many factors. In some cases, the chosen drug administration technique is the only one left. In other circumstances, the patient might have a preferred way to take their medication. Some people prefer getting their medications injected rather than ingesting them. Many would rather have it the other way around. You must always administer the medication the way it is ordered, if the patient prefers a different method, ask the doctor to change the prescribed route so you are in compliance with the medication order. The following are the variables that influence how drugs are administered:

- Favorite treatments: Although the patient shouldn't choose the method of medicine administration, it's crucial to keep in mind that everyone has preferences. It is not ideal to force injections on a patient if they do not want to get them. The doctor must persuade the patient to accept the finest medicine administration technique that is now available. While it is acceptable for patients to be reluctant to accept some forms of therapy, you should help your patients comprehend the advantages of the medication that will be given to them.

- The kind of medication to be injected: The type of medicine is the second factor that affects the method of administration. Some medications can only be taken orally. For example, it is not feasible to inject a patient with medications that are only available as tablets. Some medications should not be ingested. In such a situation, injection is the most sensible mode of administration.

- The body part being treated: The technique of medicine delivery can be greatly influenced by the area of the body that is being treated. This explains why medications used topically primarily target the skin. Direct application of the medication to the eye is reasonable if a person has an eye infection.

- How the medicine works: The drug's mechanism of action is another crucial issue to take into account. Some medications act by directly destroying the relevant pathogen. Others function by increasing the body's natural defenses against pathogens in action. Drugs function essentially in many different ways. For instance, it is preferable to inject or give a drug orally when it needs to circulate throughout the circulation. The vaginal route would be quite effective for medications that target specific organs, including the genitalia.

- Patient's physical condition: The patient's physical condition must also be taken into account. Some patients are in good physical health and can administer medications by any route. The patient might not even be able to swallow the pills in some circumstances, though. The best thing to do in such a circumstance, such as when the patient is in a coma, is to inject. However, there are several circumstances in which intramuscular and subcutaneous injections could not be effective, particularly when the patient has a skin infection. The intravenous method is the only option in such a circumstance. With intravenous injections, the medication is administered directly to the bloodstream, enabling the patient to react quickly.

Summary

- Pharmacology is the study of drugs and their effects on individuals.

- CMAs need a basic understanding of accessible medicines and their impact on patients.

- Focus on drug class categories, storage techniques, and drug reactions as a CMA.

- Medications are often categorized into six classes: depressants, barbiturates, benzodiazepines, stimulants, inhalants, hallucinogens, and cannabis.

- Understand the effects, benefits, and risks associated with each drug class.

- Educate patients on responsible medication use and the importance of doctor approval.

- Depressants induce relaxation, sleepiness, and drowsiness.

- Common depressants include tricyclic antidepressants, SSRIs, atypical antidepressants, monoamine oxidase inhibitors, and SNRIs.

- Highlight the positive effects of depressants, such as reduced anxiety and insomnia control.

- Stimulants temporarily boost energy and alertness.

- Be aware of common stimulants like cocaine and amphetamines and their potential side effects, including paranoia.

- Stress the importance of safe storage and keeping stimulants away from children.

- Inhalants are drugs that can be inhaled and alter consciousness.

- Understand the risks of inhalants, including brain and kidney damage, hearing loss, and liver damage.

- Hallucinogens can induce hallucinations and affect emotions.

- Examples include mescaline, psilocybin, and LSD.

- Be aware of the risks and side effects associated with hallucinogen use.

- Cannabis, or marijuana, is commonly abused but has some medical benefits.

- Highlight the potential negative effects, such as impaired cognitive function and hallucinations.

- Proper drug storage is vital to maintain medication potency and prevent loss.

- Medications have specific storage requirements related to temperature, humidity, and light.

- Follow manufacturer instructions to ensure correct storage conditions.

- Maintain a clean environment to prevent medication damage.

- Adverse drug reactions can range from mild to severe and are unpredictable.

- Consider drug factors, genetics, patient age, health status, and polypharmacy when assessing adverse reactions.

- Allergies and idiosyncratic reactions can occur.
- The PDR is a valuable reference containing information on FDA-approved drugs.
- It includes details on drug manufacturers, dosages, adverse reactions, and more.
- CMAs should refer to the PDR when unfamiliar with a medication.
- Drug administration methods vary and depend on factors like patient preference and the type of medication.
- Common administration methods include oral, subcutaneous, intramuscular, vaginal, and intravenous.
- Consider patient preferences, the type of medication, the target body part, the drug mechanism, and the patient's physical condition when selecting an administration method.

CHAPTER 13

Medical Specialties

ALONG WITH PREFIXES and suffixes, you also need to master some terminology related to different medical disciplines. Medical professionals are sometimes referred to as doctors. However, there are numerous divisions and classes in the medical industry. It's critical to understand the terminology used when referring to specific groups of people in the medical community as a CMA. The terms for doctors based on their specialties are listed below.

Anesthesiologists

Doctors are experts at making a wound numb and sedating patients for surgery. For instance, if a woman needs to give birth surgically, an anesthesiologist will give the patient the appropriate dosage of anesthesia or painkiller to ensure that the patient is pain-free. Anesthesiologists are typically required to be present in operating rooms.

Cardiologists

A cardiologist is an expert in diseases of the arteries, heart, and veins. In treating illnesses like heart attacks and high blood pressure, they are professionals. If you have advanced heart problems, you may be referred to a cardiologist even though other doctors may be able to diagnose these disorders.

Dermatologists

A root word that refers to the skin is dermis. A dermatologist is, in other words, a physician with an extensive understanding of the skin. Dermatologists treat conditions involving the hair, nails, and skin. For common illnesses that affect the skin and hair, they are able to diagnose, treat, and suggest remedies.

Endocrinologists

The endocrine system in the body produces hormones that control different bodily activities. A physician who focuses on diagnosing and managing endocrine-related disorders is known as an endocrinologist. Diabetes, thyroid infertility, and calcium issues are just a few of the ailments they specialize in.

Gastroenterologists

The digestive system is the area of expertise for a gastroenterologist. These doctors treat stomach cancer, ulcers, acid reflux, abdominal pain, jaundice, and diarrhea.

Geriatricians

Specialists in geriatric medicine focus on treating the elderly. While not necessarily a specialization, these doctors have extensive knowledge of the factors that influence senior patients' health as well as how they respond to various drugs. Geriatric medicine experts may work at a standard hospital, an elderly care facility, or a private practice in this area.

Hematologists

Hematologists tackle illnesses and problems affecting the spleen, blood, and lymph nodes as their areas of expertise. Hematologists treat a variety of illnesses, including hemophilia, anemia, sickle cell disease, and leukemia.

Immunologists/Allergists

Allergies, eczema, and asthma are among the immune-related disorders that these specialists address. Additionally, they test for allergies and encourage the body's immune system.

Specialists in Infectious Diseases

Specialists in infectious diseases offer prevention and treatment for diseases like HIV/AIDS, pneumonia, TB, and COVID-19. They are also experts in stopping the transmission of disease.

Internists

Internists are doctors who specialize in treating internal organs. The heart, kidneys, lungs, digestive system, and joints are the primary organs that internists care for.

Medical Geneticists

Medical geneticists are experts in treating diseases that are inherited genetically. Parents transmit these ailments to their offspring, including grandchildren. Geneticists can identify and treat genetic abnormalities that parents have handed down to their children, enabling them to lead normal lives.

Neurologists

A neurologist is a medical professional who treats nervous system disorders. They primarily deal with conditions affecting the spinal cord, brain, autonomic nervous system, cranial blood vessels, and peripheral nerves. They also cope with Parkinson's disease, convulsions, and stroke.

Obstetricians/Gynecologists

A gynecologist focuses on the female reproductive system. Gynecologists provide a wide range of tasks for their employers, including cancer, general maternal health care, and, in some cases, surgical procedures. A gynecologist treats a variety of health issues, including infertility, pelvic medicine, and womb reconstruction surgery. Obstetricians focus mostly on pregnancies and deliveries.

Ophthalmologists

An expert who treats eye conditions is known as an ophthalmologist. Ophthalmologists perform a wide range of tasks, from eye exams to eye surgery. These medical professionals deal with issues including strabismus and diabetic retinopathy.

Otolaryngologists

They are specialists in treating disorders affecting the nose, ear, throat, and sinuses and are also referred to as ENT doctors. Additionally, they might take care of neck and upper respiratory tract-related health issues. To treat abnormalities of the face and neck, certain ENTs also undertake plastic and reconstructive procedures.

Pathologists are professionals who examine tissue samples to make diagnoses. They use many different techniques, such as autopsies and biopsies, to primarily diagnose and track diseases.

Pediatricians

These clinicians specialize in caring for young patients from infancy to puberty. They mostly deal with ailments that affect kids frequently, like allergies, asthma, and croup. Pediatricians can, however, treat a wide range of other childhood conditions, including those related to growth, development, nutrition, etc.

Plastic Surgeons

Repairing damaged bodily parts is a plastic surgeon's area of expertise. The goal of the plastic surgeon is to make the organs and tissues look better and function better. They also discuss the appearance of the hands, breasts, chest, and general skin.

Psychiatrists

A psychiatrist treats ailments of the mind and the soul. Psychiatrists have received training in the relationship between a person's emotional and mental health. There are many subspecialties within this branch of psychiatry, including forensic, addiction, and general psychiatry.

The majority of CMAs will wind up collaborating with surgeons and supporting them throughout a variety of surgical operations. Listed are some of the most commonly done surgical specialties and what they actually entail.

- Abdominoplasty: To change the shape of the abdomen, this operation is performed. This treatment, which is primarily known as a tummy tuck, has grown in popularity among those who want to lose belly fat. The treatment is frequently used to treat problems caused by obesity.

- Amputation: Amputation is when a portion of a limb is removed. Amputations are typically performed to stop the spread of fatal infections. A patient's willingness to endure a vital surgical surgery like an amputation depends entirely on that patient.

- Appendectomy: The appendix is removed during an appendectomy, a surgical surgery if it is infected or inflamed. Appendicectomy is another name for the procedure.

- Breast augmentation: Breast augmentation is a surgical technique used to enhance the breasts' appearance. Under the breast muscles, silicone shells are placed during the procedure. Two main goals can be achieved with this procedure: enlarging the breast and reconstructing the breast following cancer or injury surgery.

- Gastric bypass surgery: This operation makes the stomach smaller. The patient is primarily helped with weight loss by it. Obese people typically have this kind of surgery done.

Summary

- Understanding Medical Specialties: In the medical field, there are numerous specialties, each focusing on specific areas of healthcare and diseases.

- Anesthesiologists: These specialists administer anesthesia and sedation to patients undergoing surgical procedures, ensuring they are pain-free during surgery.

- Cardiologists: Cardiologists are experts in diagnosing and treating conditions related to the heart, arteries, and veins, including heart attacks and high blood pressure.
- Dermatologists: They specialize in skin, hair, and nail conditions diagnoses and treatment.
- Endocrinologists: These specialists focus on disorders of the endocrine system, which involves hormone production and regulation, including conditions like diabetes and thyroid disorders.
- Gastroenterologists: Gastroenterologists specialize in treating disorders of the digestive system, including stomach cancer, ulcers, and acid reflux.
- Geriatricians: Geriatric medicine experts focus on the healthcare needs of elderly patients, understanding the unique factors affecting their health and medication responses.
- Hematologists: Hematologists treat disorders related to the blood, spleen, and lymph nodes, such as anemia, leukemia, and hemophilia.
- Immunologists/Allergists: These specialists address immune-related disorders, including allergies, eczema, and asthma, and can conduct allergy testing.
- Specialists in Infectious Diseases: Infectious disease specialists focus on preventing and treating diseases caused by pathogens like HIV/AIDS, pneumonia, and COVID-19.

Conclusion

AS WE CLOSE the book on this complete guide to the Certified Medical Assistant (CMA) certification, you will have a thorough understanding of what it takes to be a top-tier CMA. The terrain of medical aid is varied and multifaceted, necessitating an optimal balance of expertise, dexterity, and professionalism. We hope that this guide has instilled in you not just the ability but also the enthusiasm required to thrive in this sector.

Our investigation of the medical world has shown the broad and complex tasks that await you as a CMA, from clinical workflow to pharmacology, safety, infection control, medical regulations, and ethics. It's an extraordinary journey in which every day offers the chance to make a major difference in the lives of patients and their families.

The healthcare industry is a constantly changing ecology that necessitates a persistent need for knowledge. This book has illuminated the key duties and responsibilities you'll assume as a CMA, as well as the critical soft skills required for success, such as communication and empathy. Remember that while technical skills will get you in the door, soft skills will keep you there.

Our coverage of regulatory rules, as well as legal and ethical concerns, serves as a help in navigating the frequently complex healthcare legal landscape. These rules are more than just laws or recommendations; they are the standards that protect the healthcare profession's integrity.

We've included a number of practice exercises, ranging from clinical procedures to billing and coding, to help you solidify your understanding and assess your readiness for the CMA exam. These questions, albeit difficult, provide a look into the breadth and depth of the CMA exam and are intended to boost your confidence as you begin your certification path.

Finally, we talked about how important health information management and appointment scheduling are. Effective health information management is not only a must in today's healthcare system; it is a lifeline that maintains the smooth operation of healthcare institutions.

This book represents the end of your journey to become a Certified Medical Assistant, but it's also just the beginning in many respects. Remember that every patient encounter, every lab result, and every scheduled appointment contributes to your growth as a healthcare professional and enriches the lives of the people you serve.

As you put this book down, have an open mind to the unlimited possibilities. We hope you find this book to be an invaluable resource as you prepare for the CMA exam and throughout your healthcare career. Becoming a CMA is more than simply a title; it represents a dedication to service, excellence, and lifelong learning.

Welcome to the gratifying and exciting world of medical aid! Here's to a future in which every patient you meet benefits from your abilities, knowledge, and passion for this important profession.

Sample Questionnaire

Questions

1. What is the purpose of the CMA Exam?
   a. To test general knowledge
   b. To assess administrative skills only
   c. To evaluate clinical skills only
   d. To confirm the clinical and administrative knowledge of medical assistants

2. How many sections is the CMA Exam divided into?
   a. Two
   b. Three
   c. Four
   d. Five

3. Which of the following is NOT one of the sections of the CMA Exam?
   a. General knowledge
   b. Administrative knowledge
   c. Professional behavior
   d. Surgical procedures

4. What does the Administrative section of the CMA Exam assess?
   a. Knowledge of medical procedures
   b. Patient care skills
   c. Ability to manage medical office tasks
   d. Clinical pharmacology knowledge

5. Which section of the CMA Exam evaluates hands-on patient care skills?
   a. General knowledge
   b. Administrative knowledge
   c. Clinical knowledge

    d.   Professional behavior

6.   What is the primary purpose of the General knowledge section of the CMA Exam?
    a.   Assess communication skills
    b.   Evaluate knowledge of medical procedures
    c.   Test knowledge of medical terminology and anatomy
    d.   Focus on ethical behavior

7.   What term is used to describe the study of the structure of the human body?
    a.   Pathology
    b.   Physiology
    c.   Anatomy
    d.   Pharmacology

8.   Which of the following is NOT one of the major systems of the human body?
    a.   Muscular
    b.   Skeletal
    c.   Endocrine
    d.   Genetic

9.   What aspect of pharmacology investigates how drugs are absorbed, distributed, metabolized, and removed from the body?
    a.   Pharmacokinetics
    b.   Pharmacodynamics
    c.   Drug classification
    d.   Drug administration

10. What is the study of how medications affect the body called?
    a.   Pharmacokinetics
    b.   Pharmacodynamics
    c.   Drug classification
    d.   Drug administration

11. Which of the following is NOT one of the "Five Rights" of pharmaceutical administration?
    a. The appropriate patient
    b. The correct diagnosis
    c. The correct dose
    d. The correct route
    e. The correct time

12. What does the pathology study?
    a. The structure of the human body
    b. The effects of drugs on the body
    c. The causes and consequences of diseases
    d. The communication skills of medical assistants

13. What are the cardinal indications of inflammation?
    a. Fever, fatigue, dizziness
    b. Heat, redness, swelling, pain, and loss of function
    c. Nausea, vomiting, diarrhea
    d. Headache, blurred vision, muscle weakness

14. What is the primary reason for studying medical terminology?
    a. To communicate effectively with patients
    b. To perform surgical procedures
    c. To understand legal elements of medicine
    d. To assess clinical pharmacology

15. What part of a medical term typically denotes a body part or condition?
    a. Prefix
    b. Suffix
    c. Root word
    d. Abbreviation

16. What is the primary function of prefixes in medical terminology?
    a. To add specificity to the term

b. To denote the primary body part

c. To indicate a medical condition

d. To abbreviate the term

17. Which of the following is NOT an aspect of pharmacology knowledge?

a. Drug names

b. Drug side effects

c. Drug administration

d. Dental procedures

18. Why is understanding pharmacology important for medical assistants?

a. It helps with performing surgery.

b. It aids in understanding legal aspects of medicine.

c. It improves patient care and safety regarding medications.

d. It focuses on administrative tasks.

19. What does pharmacodynamics study?

a. How drugs are absorbed and distributed

b. The effects of drugs on the body

c. The structure of the human body

d. The diagnosis of diseases

20. What is the fundamental principle of pharmaceutical safety?

a. Prescribing the highest dose possible

b. Following the "Five Rights" of medication administration

c. Administering drugs without patient consent

d. Keeping medication information confidential

21. Which of the following is an example of an analgesic drug used for pain relief?

a. Penicillin

b. Ciprofloxacin

c. Metformin

d. Ibuprofen

22. What organization governs the regulation of prescription medications in the United States?

    a. CDC

    b. DEA

    c. FDA

    d. WHO

23. How is medication absorption affected by end-stage liver disease?

    a. Enhanced absorption

    b. No impact on absorption

    c. Reduced absorption

    d. Accelerated metabolism

24. What is the purpose of the six rights of medication administration?

    a. To ensure patient comfort

    b. To prevent medication contamination

    c. To enhance medication absorption

    d. To ensure pharmaceutical safety

25. Which of the following is an example of a vaccine?

    a. Lisinopril

    b. Albuterol

    c. Influenza vaccine

    d. Loratadine

26. Which route of medication administration involves inserting drugs in the rectum?

    a. Oral

    b. Intramuscular

    c. Rectal

    d. Inhalation

27. What should you do before administering an intramuscular injection to prevent injection into a blood vessel?

    a. Apply a tourniquet

b. Massage the injection site

c. Aspirate the syringe

d. Use a larger needle gauge

28. What is the standard unit for measuring liquid medications?
    a. Milligrams (mg)
    b. Milliliters (ml)
    c. Micrograms (mcg)
    d. Centimeters (cm)

29. Which medication administration route has the fastest onset of action?
    a. Oral
    b. Subcutaneous
    c. Inhalation
    d. Topical

30. What medication is commonly used as a blood thinner?
    a. Levothyroxine
    b. Naproxen
    c. Warfarin
    d. Glipizide

31. What is the primary purpose of packaging medications properly?
    a. To reduce medication cost
    b. To improve patient compliance
    c. To prevent medication contamination
    d. To extend medication shelf life

32. Which of the following is an example of an antihypertensive medication?
    a. Metformin
    b. Oxycodone
    c. Lisinopril
    d. Sertraline

33. In which organization's guidelines should medical assistants be well-informed regarding the disposal of medications?

    a.   CDC

    b.   DEA

    c.   WHO

    d.   FDA

34. What medication administration route involves the use of an inhaler?

    a.   Intramuscular

    b.   Oral

    c.   Inhalation

    d.   Sublingual

35. Which of the following is an example of an antipsychotic medication?

    a.   Metoprolol

    b.   Omeprazole

    c.   Risperidone

    d.   Liraglutide

36. How many rights of medication administration are there?

    a.   Three

    b.   Four

    c.   Five

    d.   Six

37. What is the primary purpose of reconstituting medications in saline or water?

    a.   To increase shelf life

    b.   To reduce medication cost

    c.   To facilitate administration

    d.   To enhance medication absorption

38. Which medication is commonly used to treat thyroid disorders?

    a.   Warfarin

b. Insulin

c. Levothyroxine

d. Metformin

39. What is the preferred site for intramuscular injections in adults?

a. Buttocks

b. Thigh

c. Upper arm

d. Deltoid muscle

40. How should medical assistants dispose of needles and syringes?

a. In regular trash bins

b. In sharps containers

c. By flushing them down the toilet

d. By burying them in the ground

41. What is the primary responsibility of a medical assistant in the administrative role?

a. Assisting with surgeries

b. Managing patient records

c. Providing direct patient care

d. Conducting laboratory tests

42. What does a medical receptionist primarily focus on?

a. Assisting with medical procedures

b. Handling billing and insurance claims

c. Managing patient appointments and records

d. Providing direct patient care

43. Why is efficient scheduling important in healthcare?

a. It reduces wait times for patients

b. It maximizes revenue for the practice

c. It minimizes the need for medical records

d. It decreases patient visits

44. What does HIPAA stand for?
    a. Healthcare Insurance Payment Accountability Act
    b. Health Information Privacy and Portability Act
    c. Health Insurance Portability and Accountability Act
    d. Healthcare Information Protection and Accountability Act

45. Which of the following tasks is NOT typically handled by a medical receptionist?
    a. Managing patient appointments
    b. Handling insurance claims
    c. Coordinating communication within the facility
    d. Administering medications to patients

46. What role does a Patient Navigator/Advocate play in healthcare?
    a. Conducting medical research
    b. Navigating patients through the healthcare system
    c. Performing surgical procedures
    d. Managing patient records

47. What is the primary focus of care coordination by a Patient Navigator/Advocate?
    a. Managing patient appointments
    b. Providing direct patient care
    c. Coordinating treatment plans and specialist appointments
    d. Billing and insurance processing

48. What is the key role of a Patient Navigator/Advocate?
    a. Administering medications
    b. Managing the facility's finances
    c. Bridging the gap between patients and the healthcare system
    d. Conducting laboratory tests

49. What is one of the primary goals of medical business practices in healthcare?
    a. Reducing patient wait times
    b. Maximizing insurance claims

    c.   Minimizing the role of electronic health records

    d.   Streamlining healthcare provider duties

50. Why is understanding medical coding and billing important for CMAs?

    a.   To perform surgeries

    b.   To handle insurance claims and billing

    c.   To assist with laboratory tests

    d.   To manage patient records

51. What role does electronic health records (EHRs) play in healthcare administration?

    a.   Reducing patient appointments

    b.   Increasing paper usage

    c.   Improving communication among healthcare providers

    d.   Decreasing patient privacy

52. What is the primary source of information for healthcare practitioners about a patient's medical history and treatment?

    a.   Insurance claims

    b.   Medical billing

    c.   Patient's medical record

    d.   Laboratory test results

53. Which law governs the privacy and security of patient information in healthcare?

    a.   Medical Information Privacy Act (MIPA)

    b.   Patient Confidentiality Act (PCA)

    c.   Health Insurance Portability and Accountability Act (HIPAA)

    d.   Healthcare Privacy and Security Act (HPSA)

54. What does care coordination involve in healthcare?

    a.   Coordinating communication within the facility

    b.   Managing practice finances

    c.   Navigating patients through the healthcare system

    d.   Handling laboratory tests

55. What role does a well-organized scheduling system play in healthcare?
    a. Increasing worker productivity
    b. Maximizing wait times for patients
    c. Reducing the need for healthcare providers
    d. Decreasing patient records' quality

56. How do Electronic Health Records (EHRs) benefit healthcare practices?
    a. They decrease patient privacy
    b. They reduce the need for medical coding
    c. They improve communication among healthcare providers
    d. They increase patient billing errors

57. Why is understanding healthcare rules and regulations important for CMAs?
    a. To reduce patient appointments
    b. To provide direct patient care
    c. To ensure patient privacy and ethical practice
    d. To maximize revenue for the practice

58. What is the primary goal of medical record administration in healthcare?
    a. To reduce healthcare provider communication
    b. To improve patient billing
    c. To decrease the quality of care provided
    d. To provide effective, personalized care

59. What does managing practice finances entail for a Certified Medical Assistant (CMA)?
    a. Administering medications to patients
    b. Coordinating care between healthcare providers
    c. Handling insurance claims, billing, and financial reporting
    d. Navigating patients through the healthcare system

60. How can efficient scheduling benefit a medical practice?
    a. By maximizing wait times for patients
    b. By increasing worker productivity

    c.   By decreasing patient billing errors

    d.   By reducing the need for medical records

61.   How are scheduling and finances interconnected in a healthcare practice?

    a.   They are entirely separate concepts.

    b.   Effective scheduling can improve financial efficiency.

    c.   Finances have no impact on scheduling.

    d.   Scheduling has no effect on financial health.

62.   Which of the following is a way that proper scheduling can benefit a healthcare practice financially?

    a.   Increasing no-shows and cancellations

    b.   Reducing the need for medical equipment

    c.   Decreasing wait times for patients

    d.   Eliminating administrative tasks

63.   What is the primary role of a Certified Medical Assistant (CMA) in terms of scheduling and finances?

    a.   Managing patient records

    b.   Administering medications

    c.   Assisting with surgeries

    d.   Efficiently arranging appointments and understanding practice finances

64.   How can CMAs contribute to reducing no-shows and cancellations?

    a.   By increasing patient wait times

    b.   By maintaining disorganized schedules

    c.   By ensuring patients receive excellent treatment

    d.   By disregarding appointment reminders

65.   What is one of the critical responsibilities of a CMA in patient interaction?

    a.   Managing practice finances

    b.   Providing a welcoming environment

    c.   Handling insurance claims

d.   Conducting laboratory tests

66. What does effective communication entail for CMAs in patient interaction?
   a.   Minimizing patient questions
   b.   Keeping patient histories confidential
   c.   Providing a safe and open environment
   d.   Avoiding patient interaction

67. In which situations might CMAs assist doctors and nurses during medical procedures?
   a.   In administrative tasks only
   b.   In all clinical activities
   c.   In medical procedures as needed
   d.   In conducting laboratory tests

68. What is one of the clinical responsibilities of CMAs regarding laboratory specimens?
   a.   Managing patient appointments
   b.   Assisting with surgeries
   c.   Collecting and preparing laboratory specimens
   d.   Handling insurance claims

69. What is the purpose of conducting basic laboratory tests in healthcare settings?
   a.   To reduce patient wait times
   b.   To improve patient billing
   c.   To streamline healthcare provider duties
   d.   To properly manage patients

70. What is a critical consideration when CMAs administer medications?
   a.   Maximizing revenue for the practice
   b.   Understanding the medications' purposes, doses, and potential side effects
   c.   Coordinating communication within the facility
   d.   Reducing laboratory tests

71. What role does patient education play in a CMA's responsibilities?

    a. Managing practice finances

    b. Administering medications

    c. Advising patients on medication, lifestyle changes, and follow-up treatment

    d. Conducting laboratory tests

72. Why is infection control and safety measures crucial for CMAs?

    a. To increase patient wait times

    b. To reduce laboratory costs

    c. To provide a safe healthcare environment

    d. To eliminate patient interactions

73. What makes the clinical role of a CMA dynamic and varied?

    a. Focusing only on pediatric care

    b. The type of medical practice and state legislation

    c. Administering medications exclusively

    d. Specializing in geriatrics

74. What is the foundation of a successful patient interview for a CMA?

    a. Focusing on medical history only

    b. Empathy and excellent communication skills

    c. Asking only close-ended questions

    d. Avoiding patient interaction

75. What is the primary goal of interviewing a patient's past medical history?

    a. Determining chronic illnesses

    b. Avoiding discussion of lifestyle behaviors

    c. Focusing on the patient's immediate symptoms

    d. Excluding information about allergies

76. What is an essential part of examination room techniques for CMAs?

    a. Preparing the examination room after each patient

    b. Ignoring the patient's condition

c. Using excessive medical equipment

d. Wearing personal protective equipment

77. Why is proper wound care knowledge important for CMAs?

   a. To minimize patient interaction

   b. To provide excellent patient care

   c. To focus on administrative tasks

   d. To increase patient wait times

78. What is the primary goal of emergency management for CMAs?

   a. Increasing treatment time

   b. Assessing and responding to emergencies swiftly and appropriately

   c. Avoiding communication with healthcare professionals

   d. Administering medications during emergencies

79. Why is basic first aid important for CMAs?

   a. To replace the role of healthcare professionals

   b. To stabilize patients until advanced medical therapy is available

   c. To conduct advanced medical procedures

   d. To increase patient wait times

80. What is a critical aspect of patient education and communication for CMAs?

   a. Minimizing communication with patients

   b. Notifying patients about their care

   c. Ignoring patients' concerns

   d. Avoiding communication with healthcare providers

81. What is one of the most critical aspects of patient education for CMAs?

   a. Administrative tasks

   b. Medication instruction

   c. Laboratory specimen collection

   d. Infection control measures

82. What does effective patient education aim to achieve?
    a. Minimizing patient involvement in their care
    b. Reducing patient satisfaction
    c. Empowering patients to make informed decisions
    d. Limiting communication with patients

83. What is the primary goal of cultural competence in healthcare?
    a. Reducing patient engagement
    b. Ignoring cultural differences
    c. Improving communication and trust
    d. Avoiding diverse patient populations

84. Which of the following is NOT one of the cornerstones of effective communication?
    a. Clarity
    b. Respect
    c. Patience
    d. Active listening

85. Why is clarity important in effective communication?
    a. It includes medical jargon
    b. It simplifies information for patients
    c. It confuses patients
    d. It discourages questions

86. What is the "teach-back" method in communication?
    a. Teaching patients to become healthcare providers
    b. Asking patients to describe information in their own words
    c. Ignoring patient questions
    d. Encouraging patients to stay silent

87. How can CMAs enhance non-verbal communication?
    a. Use complex medical terminology
    b. Maintain eye contact and open body language

  c. Avoid all non-verbal cues

  d. Speak quickly

88. What is the role of a CMA regarding the Health Insurance Portability and Accountability Act (HIPAA)?

  a. Violate patient confidentiality

  b. Ignore HIPAA regulations

  c. Protect patient privacy and confidentiality

  d. Over-share patient information

89. What should CMAs do to ensure cultural competence in healthcare?

  a. Promote their own culture above others

  b. Avoid seeking input from patients of different cultures

  c. Learn about cultural beliefs and practices

  d. Use medical jargon to communicate with all patients

90. What is the first step in developing cultural competence?

  a. Speaking louder to overcome language barriers

  b. Self-reflection and awareness

  c. Using medical terminology to impress patients

  d. Ignoring cultural differences

91. What is the primary purpose of patient education for CMAs?

  a. To limit patient involvement in their care

  b. To ensure patients remain uninformed

  c. To empower patients to make informed decisions

  d. To increase patient anxiety

92. How can CMAs accommodate different learning styles in patient education?

  a. Use only written materials

  b. Utilize a variety of instructional approaches

  c. Avoid patient engagement

  d. Rely solely on verbal communication

93. What is breach?
    a. An act of gaining trust
    b. An act of spreading facts
    c. An act of breaking or failing to fulfill a promise
    d. A breach is when PHI is obtained, accessed, used, or disclosed in a way that is against the Privacy Rule.

94. What is the primary goal of legal boundaries in a CMA's scope of practice?
    a. To encourage CMAs to exceed their roles
    b. To limit patient care
    c. To define the tasks and responsibilities of CMAs
    d. To prevent CMAs from seeking further education

95. Why is it essential for CMAs to respect patient privacy and confidentiality?
    a. To limit patient trust
    b. To comply with HIPAA regulations
    c. To discourage patients from seeking medical care
    d. To speed up healthcare processes

96. Which of the following is NOT a cornerstone of effective communication?
    a. Clarity
    b. Empathy
    c. Incomplete information
    d. Active listening

97. How can CMAs overcome communication barriers in healthcare?
    a. Avoid involving interpreters
    b. Use medical jargon extensively
    c. Utilize plain language and medical interpreters
    d. Speak loudly and quickly

98. What should CMAs consider when tailoring patient education materials to individuals?
    a. One-size-fits-all approach

b. Cultural beliefs and practices

c. Patient age only

d. Avoid patient preferences

99. Why is cultural competence important in healthcare?

a. To promote cultural insensitivity

b. To limit diversity in healthcare settings

c. To improve communication and trust with diverse patients

d. To encourage cultural bias

100. What does cultural humility entail?

a. Ignoring cultural differences

b. Recognizing one's own cultural limitations

c. Promoting cultural biases

d. Excluding diverse patients from care

101. What ethical principle emphasizes a patient's right to make their healthcare decisions?

a. Nonmaleficence

b. Beneficence

c. Patient autonomy

d. Confidentiality

102. Informed consent in healthcare entails:

a. Protecting patient privacy

b. Describing procedures, potential dangers, and benefits to patients

c. Avoiding harm to patients

d. Ensuring patient confidentiality

103. What is the core principle of nonmaleficence in healthcare ethics?

a. Protecting patient privacy

b. Respecting patient autonomy

c. Avoiding harm to the patient

d. Ensuring informed consent

104. Which of the following is NOT a core ethical concept in healthcare?

    a. Beneficence

    b. Nonmaleficence

    c. Justice

    d. Competition

105. When healthcare professionals face ethical dilemmas, they can seek guidance from which sources?

    a. Legal obligations only

    b. Personal beliefs only

    c. Institutional ethical committees, peers, and mentors

    d. Patient preferences only

106. Why is cultural competence important for healthcare professionals?

    a. To avoid legal issues

    b. To provide quality patient care and respect patients' diverse backgrounds

    c. To increase competition among healthcare providers

    d. To enforce federal regulations

107. Which federal regulation protects patients' privacy by limiting how medical information is stored, exchanged, and accessed?

    a. The Occupational Safety and Health Administration (OSHA)

    b. The Health Insurance Portability and Accountability Act (HIPAA)

    c. The Centers for Disease Control and Prevention (CDC)

    d. The Food and Drug Administration (FDA)

108. What is the primary role of the Occupational Safety and Health Administration (OSHA) in healthcare?

    a. Regulating medical billing and coding

    b. Ensuring healthcare affordability

    c. Enforcing workplace safety, including infection control standards

    d. Administering healthcare insurance programs

109. Why is it important for healthcare professionals to understand state-specific patient privacy laws in addition to HIPAA?

    a. To protect patient health records

    b. To ensure proper billing and coding

    c. To enforce federal regulations

    d. To prioritize competition among healthcare providers

110. Which professional organization provides a Code of Ethics and Creed for healthcare professionals to follow?

    a. Centers for Disease Control and Prevention (CDC)

    b. Occupational Safety and Health Administration (OSHA)

    c. American Association of Medical Assistants (AAMA)

    d. Food and Drug Administration (FDA)

111. What is the primary purpose of infection control guidelines provided by the Centers for Disease Control and Prevention (CDC)?

    a. Ensuring fair billing practices

    b. Regulating drug manufacturing

    c. Preventing the spread of infectious diseases in healthcare settings

    d. Enforcing workplace safety standards

112. Why is continuing education important for healthcare professionals?

    a. It is not required for certification renewal.

    b. It keeps professionals up-to-date on legal, ethical, and professional standards.

    c. It focuses solely on clinical skills improvement.

    d. It is primarily for physicians, not healthcare professionals.

113. What is the primary goal of medical law?

    a. To ensure healthcare services are cost-effective

    b. To guarantee that healthcare services are safe, efficient, and ethical

    c. To prioritize competition among healthcare providers

    d. To administer healthcare insurance programs

114. What constitutes medical malpractice?
    a.   Providing substandard care
    b.   Overcharging patients
    c.   Offering alternative treatment options
    d.   Dispensing prescriptions

115. What is the primary purpose of informed consent in healthcare?
    a.   To protect healthcare providers from liability
    b.   To ensure patients are aware of all medical procedures
    c.   To explain the benefits of treatment to patients
    d.   To allow patients to make informed decisions about their care

116. Which ethical principle encourages healthcare professionals to take actions that benefit patients?
    a.   Autonomy
    b.   Beneficence
    c.   Nonmaleficence
    d.   Confidentiality

117. What does the principle of autonomy in healthcare emphasize?
    a.   Treating all patients equitably
    b.   Protecting patient privacy
    c.   Respecting patients' capacity to make informed decisions
    d.   Avoiding harm to patients

118. In healthcare, what does the principle of justice refer to?
    a.   Prioritizing the wealthy patients
    b.   Treating all patients equitably
    c.   Avoiding harm to patients
    d.   Providing treatment only to patients with insurance

119. Which ethical concept emphasizes the importance of keeping patient medical information private?

   a.   Autonomy

   b.   Beneficence

   c.   Nonmaleficence

   d.   Confidentiality

120. What is the primary role of the pituitary gland in the endocrine system?

   a.   Production of digestive enzymes

   b.   Production of hormones for growth and development

   c.   Regulation of sleep patterns

   d.   Detoxification of the body

121. What is the primary function of the respiratory system?

   a.   To regulate body temperature

   b.   To filter toxins from the blood

   c.   To deliver oxygen to the blood

   d.   To digest food

122. Which of the following organs is not part of the lower respiratory system?

   a.   Trachea

   b.   Bronchus

   c.   Pharynx

   d.   Lungs

123. How many lobes does the right lung have?

   a.   One

   b.   Two

   c.   Three

   d.   Four

124. What is the primary role of the kidneys in the urinary system?
    a. Producing red blood cells
    b. Balancing body fluids
    c. Aiding in digestion
    d. Regulating body temperature

125. How many nephrons are there in each kidney, on average?
    a. 100
    b. 500
    c. 1,000
    d. 10,000

126. Which hormone regulates salt reabsorption in the kidneys?
    a. Aldosterone
    b. Insulin
    c. Estrogen
    d. Testosterone

127. What is the primary function of the female reproductive system?
    a. Producing sperm
    b. Generating egg cells
    c. Filtering waste from the body
    d. Regulating blood pressure

128. Which female reproductive organ houses the fertilized egg until it becomes a baby?
    a. Vagina
    b. Ovaries
    c. Uterus
    d. Fallopian tubes

129. What are the external female reproductive organs?
    a. Vagina and uterus
    b. Labia minora and labia majora

    c.   Ovaries and fallopian tubes

    d.   Cervix and clitoris

130. Which male accessory glands produce fluids required by the male reproductive system?

    a.   Testicles

    b.   Vas deferens

    c.   Vesicles and prostate glands

    d.   Urethra

131. What is the primary function of the integumentary system?

    a.   Producing hormones

    b.   Facilitating digestion

    c.   Protecting, supporting, and aiding in body mobility

    d.   Filtering blood

132. What is the outermost layer of the skin called?

    a.   Dermis

    b.   Hypodermis

    c.   Epidermis

    d.   Subcutis

133. Which skin lesion is characterized by a raised, spherical shape with a diameter of less than 0.5 cm?

    a.   Macule

    b.   Patch

    c.   Papule

    d.   Nodule

134. What skin disorder is characterized by itching and dry skin after contact with an irritant?

    a.   Hemangioma

    b.   Melanoma

    c.   Xerosis

    d.   Contact dermatitis

135. Which patient position involves lying on the back with the head and upper body elevated at an angle of 45 to 60 degrees?
    a.   Prone
    b.   Trendelenburg
    c.   Supine
    d.   Fowler

136. In which patient position is the patient lying on the abdomen with the back to the ceiling, often used in neck or back surgery?
    a.   Prone
    b.   Supine
    c.   Trendelenburg
    d.   Lithotomy

137. What should be assessed before placing a patient in any surgical position?
    a.   Patient's age
    b.   Patient's skin condition
    c.   Patient's weight
    d.   All of the above

138. Which hormone is responsible for the development of male sexual characteristics?
    a.   Estrogen
    b.   Progesterone
    c.   Testosterone
    d.   LH

139. What is the primary function of the urethra in both males and females?
    a.   Transporting urine from the kidneys to the bladder
    b.   Transporting sperm from the testicles to the penis
    c.   Regulating blood pressure
    d.   Facilitating digestion

140. Which organ secretes the hormone aldosterone, regulating salt reabsorption from renal tubules?

    a.   Liver

    b.   Kidneys

    c.   Adrenal gland

    d.   Pancreas

141. What term describes the patient's front side?

    a.   Dorsal

    b.   Inferior

    c.   Anterior

    d.   Posterior

142. Which plane divides the body into left and right sides?

    a.   Sagittal

    b.   Frontal

    c.   Transverse

    d.   Median

143. What is the term for a muscle's attachment point that moves when the muscle contracts?

    a.   Origin

    b.   Belly

    c.   Tendon

    d.   Insertion

144. Which movement term describes drawing an organ away from the body's midline?

    a.   Abduction

    b.   Adduction

    c.   Rotation

    d.   Flexion

145. What skin disorder causes white patches on the skin due to melanocyte loss?

    a.   Psoriasis

    b.   Vitiligo

    c.   Rosacea

    d.   Eczema

146. Which heart condition involves the weakening of heart muscles, leading to organ failure?

    a.   Arrhythmia

    b.   Cardiomyopathy

    c.   Coronary Artery Disease

    d.   Pericarditis

147. What diagnostic method is used to examine the electrical pathways of the heart?

    a.   X-ray

    b.   MRI

    c.   CT scan

    d.   ECG/EKG

148. Which lead configuration is commonly used for a 12-lead ECG?

    a.   One lead

    b.   Four leads

    c.   Six leads

    d.   Twelve leads

149. What aspect of the ECG measures the regularity of the cardiac cycle?

    a.   Rate

    b.   Rhythm

    c.   Axis

    d.   Hypertrophy

150. Which medical professionals can perform an ECG?

    a.   Only doctors

    b.   Nurses and doctors

    c.   Doctors and physician assistants

    d.   Nurses, medical assistants, doctors, and physician assistants

151. What condition involves inflammation of the pericardium, the membrane around the heart?
    a. Angina pectoris
    b. Pericarditis
    c. Myocardial ischemia
    d. Cardiomyopathy

152. How many leads are used to perform a standard 12-lead ECG?
    a. 6 leads
    b. 8 leads
    c. 10 leads
    d. 12 leads

153. What is the term for a movement that draws a bodily component towards the midline or inwards?
    a. Abduction
    b. Adduction
    c. Flexion
    d. Extension

154. Which type of arthritis is associated with skin patches and is only seen in individuals with psoriasis?
    a. Rheumatoid Arthritis
    b. Osteoarthritis
    c. Psoriatic Arthritis
    d. Gout

155. What is the primary purpose of an ECG?
    a. To make a diagnosis
    b. To assess skin health
    c. To examine the nervous system
    d. To evaluate heart health

156. Which term describes the direction of the heart's electrical conductivity?
   a. Rate
   b. Rhythm
   c. Axis
   d. Hypertrophy

157. What medical condition occurs when the spinal cord narrows, putting pressure on the nerves?
   a. Scoliosis
   b. Spinal Stenosis
   c. Osteoporosis
   d. Herniated Disc

158. Which skin condition causes painful blisters due to the immune system attacking the skin's surface?
   a. Vitiligo
   b. Bursitis
   c. Epidermolysis Bullosa
   d. Pemphigus

159. What is the primary purpose of positioning the paper in the ECG machine and setting gain and speed?
   a. To clean the machine
   b. To prepare for surgery
   c. To record the patient's history
   d. To configure the ECG for proper recording

160. Which condition involves recurrent spasms in the bladder and is more common in females?
   a. Interstitial Cystitis
   b. Urinary Tract Infection (UTI)
   c. Incontinence
   d. Prostatitis

161. What equipment is required for an EKG?

   a.   Needles and syringes

   b.   Stethoscope and blood pressure cuff

   c.   Electrodes and ECG paper

   d.   Surgical instruments

162. Which of the following is NOT used in preparing a patient for an EKG?

   a.   Gauze and skin prep solution

   b.   Electrodes

   c.   Razor and tape to remove hair

   d.   Skin adhesive

163. Which of the following is NOT an example of a pointer to learn and master ECG?

   a.   Starting with the right arm with red electrode

   b.   Using red, yellow, and green electrodes in a clockwise motion

   c.   Placing electrode V6 in the midclavicular line

   d.   Placing electrode black on the right leg

164. Where are leads V1 and V2 positioned during an EKG?

   a.   On the right and left sides of the sternum at the fourth intercostal space (ICS)

   b.   In the midaxillary line at the fifth intercostal gap

   c.   Between V4 and V6

   d.   In the anterior axillary at the fifth intercostal gap

165. What does the P wave signify in an EKG?

   a.   Ventricular contraction

   b.   Atrial contraction

   c.   Heart's state of rest

   d.   Depolarization of the ventricles

166. Which of the following is NOT a medical abbreviation?

   a.   CPR

   b.   ABC

   c.   EEG

   d.   MI

167. What does the abbreviation "AFB" stand for in medical terminology?

   a.   Away from bed

   b.   Acid fast bacilli

   c.   Atrial fibrillation

   d.   Anterior cruciate ligament

168. Which blood test measures blood sugar levels?

   a.   CBC

   b.   BUN

   c.   FBS

   d.   CK

169. Which bloodborne pathogen causes AIDS?

   a.   Zika virus

   b.   Hepatitis B

   c.   Malaria

   d.   HIV

170. What is the primary agency responsible for setting guidelines on bloodborne infections in the workplace?

   a.   CDC (Centers for Disease Control and Prevention)

   b.   FDA (Food and Drug Administration)

   c.   WHO (World Health Organization)

   d.   OSHA (Occupational Safety and Health Administration)

171. Which bodily fluids are subject to universal precautions?

   a.   Cerebrospinal fluid, sputum, and urine

   b.   Blood, semen, and vaginal discharge

   c.   Sweat, nasal secretions, and feces

   d.   Amniotic fluid, tears, and synovial fluid

172. Which agency introduced the OSHA Bloodborne Pathogens Standard?
    a. CDC
    b. FDA
    c. WHO
    d. OSHA

173. What is the primary purpose of the OSHA Bloodborne Pathogens Standard?
    a. To reduce worker exposure to airborne pathogens
    b. To improve workplace lighting conditions
    c. To enhance employee communication skills
    d. To reduce worker exposure to bloodborne diseases

174. How often should the exposure control plan be updated according to the OSHA Bloodborne Pathogens Standard?
    a. Every month
    b. Annually
    c. Every 2 years
    d. Only when there's a disease outbreak

175. Which of the following is NOT recommended by OSHA for reducing the risk of exposure to bloodborne pathogens?
    a. Providing safety gear like gloves and masks
    b. Encouraging the use of needle-free techniques
    c. Offering free post-exposure examinations
    d. Encouraging workers to handle sharps without precautions

176. What is the most common bloodborne pathogen in North America?
    a. Zika virus
    b. Hepatitis B
    c. Malaria
    d. Ebola virus

177. What type of infection can result from bloodborne pathogens?
    a. Chronic diseases only
    b. Acute diseases only
    c. Both acute and chronic diseases
    d. No diseases

178. What bodily fluids are generally least likely to spread germs according to universal precautions?
    a. Sweat and tears
    b. Sputum and urine
    c. Feces and perspiration
    d. Nasal secretions and saliva

179. Which of the following is NOT a typical bloodborne pathogen spread through blood?
    a. HIV
    b. Malaria
    c. Hepatitis C
    d. Zika virus

180. What does the abbreviation "EMG" stand for in medical terminology?
    a. Emergency Medical Group
    b. Electroencephalogram
    c. Electromyogram
    d. Endoscopic retrograde cholangiopancreatography

181. Who needs to complete bloodborne pathogen training?
    a. Only healthcare workers
    b. Only first responders
    c. Anyone susceptible to exposure to bloodborne pathogens
    d. Only doctors and nurses

182. What should you do immediately after a needlestick injury?
    a. Wait for a few hours to see if any symptoms develop

b.   Wash the affected area with soap and water

c.   Ignore it and continue working

d.   Document the incident but take no action

183. What bloodborne pathogens should you be tested for after an exposure incident?

    a.   HIV and hepatitis B

    b.   HIV and hepatitis C

    c.   Hepatitis B and tetanus

    d.   Hepatitis C and tetanus

184. What treatment is recommended for hepatitis B after an exposure incident?

    a.   Hepatitis B vaccine

    b.   Hepatitis B immune globulin and vaccine

    c.   Hepatitis B immune globulin only

    d.   No treatment is needed for hepatitis B

185. What is the main purpose of the OSHA Bloodborne Pathogens Standard?

    a.   To provide guidelines for using bloodborne pathogens in research

    b.   To reduce worker exposure to bloodborne diseases

    c.   To mandate hepatitis B vaccination for all healthcare workers

    d.   To encourage the use of needles in healthcare procedures

186. Which bodily fluids are subject to universal precautions?

    a.   Nasal secretions and feces

    b.   Blood and semen

    c.   Sweat and tears

    d.   Urine and saliva

187. What is the proper procedure for handling a choking victim?

    a.   Perform back blows and abdominal thrusts

    b.   Immediately start CPR

    c.   Encourage the victim to drink water

    d.   Apply ice to the victim's neck

188. How should you treat a minor wound that is bleeding?
    a. Apply a tourniquet above the wound
    b. Wash it with soap and water and apply an adhesive bandage
    c. Ignore it, as it will stop bleeding on its own
    d. Apply a hot compress to the wound

189. What is the recommended treatment for frostbite?
    a. Immerse the affected area in hot water
    b. Rub the area vigorously to warm it up
    c. Gradually warm the area with warm clothing or blankets
    d. Apply ice packs to the frostbitten area

190. What should you do if someone is having an asthma attack?
    a. Give them a cigarette to help them relax
    b. Immediately administer their inhaler or medication
    c. Ignore it, as it will pass on its own
    d. Perform abdominal thrusts

191. How should you treat a snakebite in a remote area before seeking medical help?
    a. Suck the venom out of the wound
    b. Apply a tourniquet above the bite
    c. Wrap a bandage tightly around the bitten limb
    d. Keep the patient calm and immobilize the bitten limb

192. What should you do if someone is experiencing a seizure?
    a. Hold them down to prevent further movement
    b. Put a wooden object in their mouth to prevent biting their tongue
    c. Loosen their clothing and protect them from nearby hazards
    d. Administer CPR immediately

193. What is the first step in providing CPR to an adult who is unresponsive?
    a. Check for a pulse
    b. Begin chest compressions

c.   Open the airway and check for breathing

d.   Perform abdominal thrusts

194. When should you use an external defibrillator on a cardiac arrest victim?

a.   Immediately after detecting unresponsiveness

b.   Only if a doctor is present

c.   After performing CPR for at least 10 minutes

d.   Only if the victim is a child

195. What should you do if you encounter a person who has been stung by an insect and is experiencing an allergic reaction?

a.   Apply a tourniquet above the sting site

b.   Administer CPR immediately

c.   Use an epinephrine auto-injector if available

d.   Ignore the reaction, as it will subside on its own

196. What is the proper way to stop bleeding from a wound?

a.   Rub the wound vigorously to promote clotting

b.   Apply a cold compress directly to the wound

c.   Elevate the injured limb above the heart

d.   Apply pressure with a clean cloth and elevate the limb

197. How should you handle a patient with a nosebleed?

a.   Have the patient tilt their head back

b.   Pinch the nostrils together and have the patient lean forward

c.   Apply ice directly to the nose

d.   Ask the patient to blow their nose forcefully

198. What is the recommended treatment for a minor insect bite or sting?

a.   Apply a tourniquet above the bite

b.   Wash the area with soap and water and apply a cold compress

c.   Ignore it, as it will stop itching on its own

d.   Apply alcohol directly to the bite

199. How should you assist a person who is experiencing cardiac arrest?
    a.   Begin CPR immediately
    b.   Administer an aspirin tablet
    c.   Have the person drink water
    d.   Wait for medical professionals to arrive

200. What is the recommended treatment for a person experiencing hypothermia?
    a.   Immerse them in hot water to warm up quickly
    b.   Give them alcoholic beverages to raise their body temperature
    c.   Gradually warm them up in a warm environment and remove wet clothing
    d.   Wrap them in a cold, wet blanket

201. What should be the immediate response when encountering a physical accident involving a joint dislocation?
    a.   Administer CPR
    b.   Apply heat to the affected joint
    c.   Assess the severity and transport the patient to a hospital if severe
    d.   Apply compression to the joint

202. Which acronym represents the first-aid method for managing small wounds, including joint dislocations, in the initial 48 hours?
    a.   CPR
    b.   RICE
    c.   ABC
    d.   AED

203. When should you administer CPR during an emergency?
    a.   When someone has a minor injury
    b.   When someone is breathing normally
    c.   When someone's heart has stopped or they are not breathing
    d.   When someone is conscious and alert

204. What is the primary goal of infection control in a healthcare setting?

   a. Reducing healthcare costs

   b. Decreasing the demand on medical facilities

   c. Preventing the spread of infectious diseases

   d. Isolating all patients with infections

205. Which of the following is NOT a recommended method for controlling infections?

   a. Mass vaccination

   b. Public health education

   c. Personal hygiene

   d. Isolation of all patients

206. What is the purpose of mass vaccination in infection control?

   a. To isolate infected patients

   b. To prevent the spread of infectious diseases

   c. To promote personal hygiene

   d. To decrease healthcare costs

207. Which method involves eliminating or drastically reducing bacteria by at least 99.9% on inanimate surfaces?

   a. Cleaning

   b. Sanitization

   c. Disinfection

   d. Sterilization

208. What is the primary distinction between sanitization and disinfection?

   a. Sanitization kills all bacteria, while disinfection eliminates only some.

   b. Sanitization focuses on removing dust and grime, while disinfection kills bacteria.

   c. Sanitization is performed before cleaning, while disinfection comes after.

   d. Sanitization requires heat, while disinfection uses chemicals.

209. Which hand hygiene method is most appropriate when hands are visibly dirty or contaminated with bodily fluids?
    a. Hand sanitizers
    b. Dry heat cabinets
    c. Alcohol-based rubs
    d. Plain soap and water

210. What is the recommended duration for washing hands with soap and water?
    a. 5 seconds
    b. 15 seconds
    c. 30 seconds
    d. 60 seconds

211. When should healthcare professionals typically wash their hands?
    a. Only after administering vaccinations
    b. Before handling medications and after leaving the aseptic area
    c. Only when hands are visibly soiled
    d. After providing first aid and not necessarily before handling medications

212. What action should be taken when there is an exposure to blood or bodily fluids during first aid?
    a. Ignore it, as it will not cause harm
    b. Wait for symptoms to develop
    c. Wash the affected area with soap and water
    d. Immediately administer CPR

213. Which of the following is NOT one of the initial actions recommended for handling an emergency?
    a. Performing CPR
    b. Scanning the area for potential danger
    c. Inspecting for bleeding
    d. Loosening clothing if necessary

214. When should you call for help during an emergency?

    a.   After performing CPR

    b.   Immediately when uncertain how to assist

    c.   Only after checking for bleeding

    d.   When all patients have been stabilized

215. In which scenario should a patient's clothing be loosened during an emergency?

    a.   When the patient is conscious and alert

    b.   When the patient has lost consciousness

    c.   When the patient is suffering from a minor injury

    d.   When the patient is seated comfortably

216. What is the primary purpose of isolating patients in a healthcare facility?

    a.   To improve patient comfort

    b.   To reduce healthcare costs

    c.   To prevent the spread of highly contagious diseases

    d.   To provide privacy to patients

217. Which government-recommended strategy can be vital in preventing the spread of infectious diseases, such as COVID-19?

    a.   Mass vaccination

    b.   Personal hygiene

    c.   Public health education

    d.   Governmental regulations

218. What is the main responsibility of CMAs in infection control?

    a.   Isolating all patients with infections

    b.   Administering vaccines

    c.   Raising public awareness

    d.   Having a fundamental knowledge of infectious agents and their management

219. Which infection control method is used to kill more than 99.99% of surface-residing bacteria?

a. Sanitization

b. Personal hygiene

c. Isolation

d. Disinfection

220. What is the primary goal of infection control in healthcare facilities?

a. Decreasing the demand on medical facilities

b. Reducing healthcare costs

c. Preventing the spread of infectious diseases

d. Isolating all patients with infections

221. Which of the following is NOT considered a major organism responsible for spreading infectious diseases?

a. Bacteria

b. Fungi

c. Parasites

d. All of the above

222. What is the primary composition of a virus?

a. DNA and RNA

b. Proteins and lipids

c. Nucleus and glycoproteins

d. Carbohydrates and fibers

223. How can the coronavirus causing COVID-19 primarily spread from one person to another?

a. Saliva interchange

b. Physical contact

c. Aerosol transmission

d. Sexual intimacy

224. Which of the following infectious agents is a living organism that depends on other living things for survival?

    a. Bacteria

    b. Viruses

    c. Fungi

    d. Parasites

225. How can parasites enter a host's body?

    a. Through physical contact only

    b. Through food and drink only

    c. Both through physical contact and food/drink

    d. Through inhalation

226. What is one of the common modes of bacterial infection transmission?

    a. Inhalation

    b. Sexual contact

    c. Ingestion

    d. Vector-borne transmission

227. Which of the following fungal infections can exist as either yeast or mold?

    a. Candida

    b. Aspergillus

    c. Histoplasma

    d. Sporothrix

228. How are infectious agents transmitted via droplet spread?

    a. Through direct physical contact

    b. Through interaction with contaminated surfaces

    c. Through microscopic droplets from coughing or sneezing

    d. Through vector-borne transmission

229. What is the main reservoir for infectious agents?

    a. Humans

    b.   Animals

    c.   Soil and water

    d.   All of the above

230. What is the primary means of transmission of infectious agents?

    a.   Direct contact

    b.   Indirect contact

    c.   Droplet spread

    d.   Vector-borne transmission

231. Which nutrient is a primary source of instant energy for the body?

    a.   Proteins

    b.   Fats

    c.   Carbohydrates

    d.   Vitamins

232. What is the main function of proteins in the body?

    a.   Providing instant energy

    b.   Supporting the growth of bones and muscles

    c.   Maintaining healthy skin and eyes

    d.   Enhancing digestion

233. Which type of fat is generally considered healthy and found in foods like olive oil and avocados?

    a.   Saturated fats

    b.   Trans fats

    c.   Monounsaturated fats

    d.   Polyunsaturated fats

234. How much protein does a healthy adult need per kilogram of body weight per day?

    a.   0.2 grams

    b.   0.4 grams

c. 0.6 grams

d. 0.8 grams

235. What is the primary composition of unsaturated fats?

a. Long-chain glucose molecules

b. Hydrogen atoms

c. Carbon, hydrogen, and oxygen

d. Fewer hydrogen atoms than saturated fats

236. Which type of carbohydrate is commonly found in vegetables, fruits, nuts, and grains and is considered healthy?

a. Starches

b. Sugars

c. Fiber

d. All carbohydrates are unhealthy

237. In infection control, what is a key step to reduce the spread of infectious agents?

a. Excessive use of antibiotics

b. Maintaining poor personal hygiene

c. Regular cleaning of personal effects

d. Ignoring waste disposal

238. Which nutrient helps in maintaining the health of the skin, teeth, and eyes?

a. Carbohydrates

b. Fats

c. Proteins

d. Vitamins

239. Which mode of infection transmission involves the use of wild and domestic animals or insects to carry infectious agents?

a. Inhalation

b. Vector-borne transmission

c. Direct contact

d.   Droplet spread

240. How can individuals reduce the risk of heart disease through dietary choices?

  a.   Consume a diet high in saturated fats

  b.   Avoid eating fish

  c.   Choose a Mediterranean diet with unsaturated fats

  d.   Eliminate carbohydrates from the diet

241. Which category of vitamins can be stored in the body for a few months?

  a.   Water-soluble vitamins

  b.   Fat-soluble vitamins

  c.   Trace minerals

  d.   Macro-minerals

242. Which vitamin is known for its role in skin health and wound healing?

  a.   Vitamin A

  b.   Vitamin B12

  c.   Vitamin C

  d.   Vitamin D

243. What vitamin is commonly found in sunlight and plays a crucial role in bone health?

  a.   Vitamin A

  b.   Vitamin B6

  c.   Vitamin D

  d.   Vitamin K

244. Which category of minerals is required by the body in relatively high amounts?

  a.   Trace minerals

  b.   Macro-minerals

  c.   Fat-soluble minerals

  d.   Water-soluble minerals

245. What is the main source of trace minerals in our diet?
   a. Fruits and vegetables
   b. Nuts and seeds
   c. Meat and poultry
   d. Whole grains

246. How many glasses of water should a healthy adult consume daily?
   a. 4 glasses
   b. 6 glasses
   c. 8 glasses
   d. 10 glasses

247. Which dietary requirement is especially important for patients with celiac disease?
   a. Weight control diet
   b. Hypertension diet
   c. Special dietary needs
   d. Cancer diet

248. Which leafy green vegetable is recommended for weight control due to its low carb and nutrient-dense nature?
   a. Kale
   b. Spinach
   c. Broccoli
   d. Swiss chard

249. What condition can result from a deficiency of water-soluble vitamins?
   a. Scurvy
   b. Rickets
   c. Beriberi
   d. Osteoporosis

250. Which health issue can be caused by the accumulation of plaque in the arteries?
    a. Osteoporosis
    b. Scurvy
    c. Hypertension
    d. Beriberi

251. Which foods are highly recommended for individuals with high blood pressure?
    a. Processed foods with added sugars
    b. Red meat
    c. Fruits
    d. Simple sugars

252. What is the primary goal of dietary recommendations for cancer patients?
    a. To induce weight loss
    b. To increase sugar intake
    c. To help regain lost mass and support healing
    d. To reduce water intake

253. What type of food is essential for cancer patients to rebuild damaged tissues?
    a. Protein-rich foods
    b. High-sugar foods
    c. High-fat foods
    d. Processed foods

254. What is the most common sugar found in dairy milk that lactose-intolerant individuals struggle to digest?
    a. Fructose
    b. Glucose
    c. Lactose
    d. Sucrose

255. Which category of drugs induces sleep and relaxation but is rarely used today due to safety concerns?
   a. Antidepressants
   b. Barbiturates
   c. Benzodiazepines
   d. Depressants

256. What is the most commonly used psychoactive substance worldwide?
   a. Cocaine
   b. Marijuana
   c. Ethanol (Alcohol)
   d. Heroin

257. Which category of drugs is commonly used to treat conditions like stress, anxiety, and insomnia?
   a. Antidepressants
   b. Barbiturates
   c. Benzodiazepines
   d. Depressants

258. What eating disorder primarily affects individuals who avoid certain foods and perceive themselves as overweight?
   a. Binge Eating
   b. Anorexia Nervosa
   c. Pica
   d. Avoidant Disorder

259. Which primary eating disorder is characterized by consuming a large amount of food all at once?
   a. Anorexia Nervosa
   b. Bulimia Nervosa
   c. Binge Eating
   d. Rumination Disorder

260. What is the main focus of pharmacological knowledge for CMAs?

    a.   Drug Class Categories

    b.   Drug Retention

    c.   Drug Reactions

    d.   All of the above

261. Which two stimulants are most frequently abused?

    a.   Marijuana and LSD

    b.   Cocaine and amphetamines

    c.   Aerosols and solvents

    d.   Psilocybin and mescaline

262. What is the most common adverse reaction to stimulant overdose?

    a.   Drowsiness

    b.   Paranoia

    c.   Nausea

    d.   Increased appetite

263. Which of the following is NOT considered an inhalant?

    a.   Spray paint

    b.   Cocaine

    c.   Gasoline

    d.   Nitrous oxide

264. What are the potential long-term impacts of inhaling chemicals regularly?

    a.   Improved cognitive function

    b.   Brain damage

    c.   Enhanced hearing

    d.   Increased kidney function

265. Which hallucinogen is naturally present in the peyote cactus?

    a.   Psilocybin

    b.   LSD

c. Cannabis

d. Mescaline

266. What is the primary motivation for recreational marijuana use?

a. Treating chronic pain

b. Reducing anxiety

c. Euphoria from THC

d. Improved cognitive function

267. What does the Physicians' Desk Reference (PDR) contain information about?

a. Cooking recipes

b. All legal medications in the US

c. Historical events

d. Famous doctors

268. Which section of the PDR contains information about a drug's manufacturer?

a. Section 1

b. Section 2

c. Section 3

d. Section 4

269. What is the most common method of drug administration?

a. Intravenous injection

b. Vaginal route

c. Oral ingestion

d. Subcutaneous injection

270. Which route of drug administration is used for insulin delivery?

a. Oral

b. Intramuscular injection

c. Subcutaneous injection

d. Vaginal route

271. Which factor does NOT influence the choice of drug administration method?
    a. Patient's preference
    b. Type of medication
    c. Patient's age
    d. Patient's blood type

272. What is the first step in proper drug storage?
    a. Checking the drug's expiration date
    b. Complying with the manufacturer's instructions
    c. Storing all drugs at room temperature
    d. Placing all drugs in direct sunlight

273. What environmental factor is crucial for storing medications?
    a. High humidity
    b. Direct sunlight
    c. Adequate lighting
    d. Extreme temperatures

274. How does proper drug storage help prevent losses?
    a. By attracting thieves
    b. By ensuring expensive items are stored securely
    c. By exposing medications to moisture
    d. By keeping medications in direct sunlight

275. Which factor primarily determines how quickly a medication is absorbed through intramuscular injection?
    a. The dosage of the medication
    b. The patient's age
    c. The blood flow in the injection area
    d. The medication's expiration date

276. What is the main purpose of the Physician's Desk Reference (PDR)?
    a. To provide medical advice

b. To list all medications used worldwide

c. To serve as a reference for doctors regarding legal medications in the US

d. To publish pharmaceutical research

277. Which section of the PDR is used for medication identification?

a. Section 1

b. Section 2

c. Section 4

d. Section 5

278. Which drug administration method delivers medication directly into the bloodstream?

a. Oral ingestion

b. Intramuscular injection

c. Subcutaneous injection

d. Intravenous (IV) administration

279. What should be considered when determining the best drug administration method?

a. Patient's preference

b. Patient's blood type

c. Medication expiration date

d. Patient's height

280. What is the typical method of administration for medications targeting the skin?

a. Intravenous injection

b. Subcutaneous injection

c. Topical application

d. Oral ingestion

281. What is the medical specialty that focuses on diseases of the arteries, heart, and veins?

a. Dermatology

b. Cardiology

c. Endocrinology

d. Ophthalmology

282. Which medical professional specializes in treating nervous system disorders?

    a.   Anesthesiologist

    b.   Neurologist

    c.   Gastroenterologist

    d.   Hematologist

283. What is the primary organ system that internists specialize in treating?

    a.   Musculoskeletal system

    b.   Respiratory system

    c.   Digestive system

    d.   Internal organs

284. What is the primary focus of a dermatologist's practice?

    a.   Heart diseases

    b.   Skin, hair, and nails

    c.   Digestive disorders

    d.   Nervous system diseases

285. Which surgical procedure is commonly performed to stop the spread of fatal infections?

    a.   Breast augmentation

    b.   Abdominoplasty

    c.   Gastric bypass surgery

    d.   Amputation

286. Who specializes in the treatment of diseases that are inherited genetically?

    a.   Immunologist

    b.   Endocrinologist

    c.   Medical geneticist

    d.   Cardiologist

287. What is the main goal of gastric bypass surgery?

    a.   To enhance breast appearance

    b.   To treat skin disorders

    c.   To reduce abdominal fat

    d.   To assist with weight loss

288. Which medical specialist is responsible for treating diseases of the digestive system?

    a.   Endocrinologist

    b.   Gastroenterologist

    c.   Cardiologist

    d.   Ophthalmologist

289. What is the primary function of an ophthalmologist?

    a.   Treating skin disorders

    b.   Diagnosing heart diseases

    c.   Treating eye conditions

    d.   Managing digestive disorders

290. What is the medical specialty focused on the elderly population?

    a.   Pediatric medicine

    b.   Geriatric medicine

    c.   Obstetrics

    d.   Psychiatry

291. Which medical specialty deals with the study of the endocrine system and related disorders?

    a.   Cardiology

    b.   Immunology

    c.   Endocrinology

    d.   Hematology

292. Which surgical procedure is commonly referred to as a "tummy tuck"?

    a.   Abdominoplasty

    b.   Breast augmentation

    c.   Gastric bypass surgery

    d.   Amputation

293. What do medical geneticists specialize in diagnosing and treating?
    a. Heart diseases
    b. Genetic disorders
    c. Skin conditions
    d. Digestive disorders

294. Which medical specialty focuses on the female reproductive system?
    a. Cardiology
    b. Ophthalmology
    c. Obstetrics/gynecology
    d. Neurology

295. What is the primary responsibility of a pathologist?
    a. Treating infectious diseases
    b. Diagnosing genetic disorders
    c. Examining tissue samples for diagnoses
    d. Performing amputations

296. What type of surgery aims to make organs and tissues look and function better?
    a. Abdominoplasty
    b. Appendectomy
    c. Plastic surgery
    d. Gastric bypass surgery

297. Who is responsible for examining and treating diseases related to the spleen, blood, and lymph nodes?
    a. Gastroenterologist
    b. Immunologist
    c. Hematologist
    d. Otolaryngologist

298. What does an infectious disease specialist primarily focus on?
    a. Heart diseases

b. Genetic disorders

c. Treating infectious diseases

d. Plastic surgery

299. Which medical professional is an expert in diagnosing and managing diseases related to allergies and the immune system?

a. Gastroenterologist

b. Immunologist/allergist

c. Endocrinologist

d. Neurologist

300. What medical specialty involves making a wound numb and sedating patients for surgery?

a. Dermatology

b. Anesthesiology

c. Geriatric medicine

d. Otolaryngology

Answers

1. d) To confirm the clinical and administrative knowledge of medical assistants

2. c) Four

3. d) Surgical procedures

4. c) Ability to manage medical office tasks

5. c) Clinical knowledge

6. c) Test knowledge of medical terminology and anatomy

7. c) Anatomy

8. d) Genetic

9. a) Pharmacokinetics

10. b) Pharmacodynamics

11. b) The correct diagnosis

12. c) The causes and consequences of diseases

13. b) Heat, redness, swelling, pain, and loss of function

14. a) To communicate effectively with patients

15. c) Root word

16. a) To add specificity to the term

17. d) Dental procedures

18. c) It improves patient care and safety regarding medications.

19. b) The effects of drugs on the body

20. b) Following the "Five Rights" of medication administration

21. d) Ibuprofen

22. c) FDA

23. c) Reduced absorption

24. d) To ensure pharmaceutical safety

25. c) Influenza vaccine

26. c) Rectal

27. c) Aspirate the syringe

28. b) Milliliters (ml)

29. c) Inhalation

30. c) Warfarin

31. c) To prevent medication contamination

32. c) Lisinopril

33. b) DEA

34. c) Inhalation

35. c) Risperidone

36. d) Six

37. c) To facilitate administration

38. c) Levothyroxine

39. a) Buttocks

40. b) In sharps containers

41. b) Managing patient records

42. c) Managing patient appointments and records

43. a) It reduces wait times for patients

44. c) Health Insurance Portability and Accountability Act

45. d) Administering medications to patients

46. b) Navigating patients through the healthcare system

47. c) Coordinating treatment plans and specialist appointments

48. c) Bridging the gap between patients and the healthcare system

49. a) Reducing patient wait times

50. b) To handle insurance claims and billing

51. c) Improving communication among healthcare providers

52. c) Patient's medical record

53. c) Health Insurance Portability and Accountability Act (HIPAA)

54. a) Coordinating communication within the facility

55. a) Increasing worker productivity

56. c) They improve communication among healthcare providers

57. c) To ensure patient privacy and ethical practice

58. d) To provide effective, personalized care

59. c) Handling insurance claims, billing, and financial reporting

60. b) By increasing worker productivity

61. b) Effective scheduling can improve financial efficiency.

62. c) Decreasing wait times for patients

63. d) Efficiently arranging appointments and understanding practice finances

64. c) By ensuring patients receive excellent treatment

65. b) Providing a welcoming environment

66. c) Providing a safe and open environment

67. c) In medical procedures as needed

68. c) Collecting and preparing laboratory specimens

69. d) To properly manage patients

70. b) Understanding the medications' purposes, doses, and potential side effects

71. c) Advising patients on medication, lifestyle changes, and follow-up treatment

72. c) To provide a safe healthcare environment

73. b) The type of medical practice and state legislation

74. b) Empathy and excellent communication skills

75. a) Determining chronic illnesses

76. a) Preparing the examination room after each patient

77. b) To provide excellent patient care

78. b) Assessing and responding to emergencies swiftly and appropriately

79. b) To stabilize patients until advanced medical therapy is available

80. b) Notifying patients about their care

81. b) Medication instruction

82. c) Empowering patients to make informed decisions

83. c) Improving communication and trust

84. c) Patience

85. b) It simplifies information for patients

86. b) Asking patients to describe information in their own words

87. b) Maintain eye contact and open body language

88. c) Protect patient privacy and confidentiality

89. c) Learn about cultural beliefs and practices

90. b) Self-reflection and awareness

91. c) To empower patients to make informed decisions

92. b) Utilize a variety of instructional approaches

93. d) A breach is when PHI is obtained, accessed, used, or disclosed in a way that is against the Privacy Rule.

94. c) To define the tasks and responsibilities of CMAs

95. b) To comply with HIPAA regulations

96. c) Incomplete information

97. c) Utilize plain language and medical interpreters

98. b) Cultural beliefs and practices

99. c) To improve communication and trust with diverse patients

100. b) Recognizing one's own cultural limitations

101. c) Patient autonomy

102. b) Describing procedures, potential dangers, and benefits to patients

103. c) Avoiding harm to the patient

104. d) Competition

105. c) Institutional ethical committees, peers, and mentors

106. b) To provide quality patient care and respect patients' diverse backgrounds

107. b) The Health Insurance Portability and Accountability Act (HIPAA)

108. c) Enforcing workplace safety, including infection control standards

109. a) To protect patient health records

110. c) American Association of Medical Assistants (AAMA)

111. c) Preventing the spread of infectious diseases in healthcare settings

112. b) It keeps professionals up-to-date on legal, ethical, and professional standards.

113. b) To guarantee that healthcare services are safe, efficient, and ethical.

114. a) Providing substandard care

115. d) To allow patients to make informed decisions about their care

116. b) Beneficence

117. c) Respecting patients' capacity to make informed decisions

118. b) Treating all patients equitably

119. d) Confidentiality

120. b) Production of hormones for growth and development

121. c) To deliver oxygen to the blood

122. c) Pharynx

123. c) Three

124. b) Balancing body fluids

125. c) 1,000

126. a) Aldosterone

127. b) Generating egg cells

128. c) Uterus

129. b) Labia minora and labia majora

130. c) Vesicles and prostate glands

131. c) Protecting, supporting, and aiding in body mobility

132. c) Epidermis

133. c) Papule

134. d) Contact dermatitis

135. d) Fowler

136. a) Prone

137. d) All of the above

138. c) Testosterone

139. a) Transporting urine from the kidneys to the bladder

140. c) Adrenal gland

141. c) Anterior

142. a) Sagittal

143. d) Insertion

144. a) Abduction

145. b) Vitiligo

146. b) Cardiomyopathy

147. d) ECG/EKG

148. d) Twelve leads

149. b) Rhythm

150. d) Nurses, medical assistants, doctors, and physician assistants

151. b) Pericarditis

152. d) 12 leads

153. b) Adduction

154. c) Psoriatic Arthritis

155. d) To evaluate heart health

156. c) Axis

157. b) Spinal Stenosis

158. d) Pemphigus

159. d) To configure the ECG for proper recording

160. a) Interstitial Cystitis

161. c) Electrodes and ECG paper

162. d) Skin adhesive

163. c) Placing electrode V6 in the midclavicular line

164. a) On the right and left sides of the sternum at the fourth intercostal space (ICS)

165. b) Atrial contraction

166. b) ABC

167. b) Acid fast bacilli

168. c) FBS

169. d) HIV

170. d) OSHA (Occupational Safety and Health Administration)

171. b) Blood, semen, and vaginal discharge

172. d) OSHA

173. d) To reduce worker exposure to bloodborne diseases

174. b) Annually

175. d) Encouraging workers to handle sharps without precautions

176. b) Hepatitis B

177. c) Both acute and chronic diseases

178. d) Nasal secretions and saliva

179. b) Malaria

180. c) Electromyogram

181. c) Anyone susceptible to exposure to bloodborne pathogens

182. b) Wash the affected area with soap and water

183. a) HIV and hepatitis B

184. b) Hepatitis B immune globulin and vaccine

185. b) To reduce worker exposure to bloodborne diseases

186. b) Blood and semen

187. a) Perform back blows and abdominal thrusts

188. b) Wash it with soap and water and apply an adhesive bandage

189. c) Gradually warm the area with warm clothing or blankets

190. b) Immediately administer their inhaler or medication

191. d) Keep the patient calm and immobilize the bitten limb

192. c) Loosen their clothing and protect them from nearby hazards

193. a) Check for a pulse

194. a) Immediately after detecting unresponsiveness

195. c) Use an epinephrine auto-injector if available

196. d) Apply pressure with a clean cloth and elevate the limb

197. b) Pinch the nostrils together and have the patient lean forward

198. b) Wash the area with soap and water and apply a cold compress

199. a) Begin CPR immediately

200. c) Gradually warm them up in a warm environment and remove wet clothing

201. c) Assess the severity and transport the patient to a hospital if severe

202. b) RICE (rest, ice, compression, and elevation)

203. c) When someone's heart has stopped or they are not breathing

204. c) Preventing the spread of infectious diseases

205. d) Isolation of all patients

206. b) To prevent the spread of infectious diseases

207. b) Sanitization

208. b) Sanitization focuses on removing dust and grime, while disinfection kills bacteria.

209. d) Plain soap and water

210. b) 15 seconds

211. b) Before handling medications and after leaving the aseptic area

212. c) Wash the affected area with soap and water

213. a) Performing CPR

214. b) Immediately when uncertain how to assist

215. b) When the patient has lost consciousness

216. c) To prevent the spread of highly contagious diseases

217. d) Governmental regulations

218. d) Having a fundamental knowledge of infectious agents and their management

219. d) Disinfection

220. c) Preventing the spread of infectious diseases

221. d) All of the above

222. b) Proteins and lipids

223. c) Aerosol transmission

224. d) Parasites

225. c) Both through physical contact and food/drink

226. c) Ingestion

227. a) Candida

228. c) Through microscopic droplets from coughing or sneezing

229. d) All of the above

230. b) Indirect contact

231. c) Carbohydrates

232. b) Supporting the growth of bones and muscles

233. c) Monounsaturated fats

234. d) 0.8 grams

235. d) Fewer hydrogen atoms than saturated fats

236. c) Fiber

237. c) Regular cleaning of personal effects

238. d) Vitamins

239. b) Vector-borne transmission

240. c) Choose a Mediterranean diet with unsaturated fats

241. b) Fat-soluble vitamins

242. c) Vitamin C

243. c) Vitamin D

244. b) Macro-minerals

245. a) Fruits and vegetables

246. c) 8 glasses

247. c) Special dietary needs

248. a) Kale

249. c) Beriberi

250. c) Hypertension

251. c) Fruits

252. c) To help regain lost mass and support healing

253. a) Protein-rich foods

254. c) Lactose

255. b) Barbiturates

256. c) Ethanol (Alcohol)

257. c) Benzodiazepines

258. b) Anorexia Nervosa

259. c) Binge Eating

260. d) All of the above

261. b) Cocaine and amphetamines

262. b) Paranoia

263. b) Cocaine

264. b) Brain damage

265. d) Mescaline

266. c) Euphoria from THC

267. b) All legal medications in the US

268. a) Section 1

269. c) Oral ingestion

270. c) Subcutaneous injection

271. d) Patient's blood type

272. b) Complying with the manufacturer's instructions

273. c) Adequate lighting

274. b) By ensuring expensive items are stored securely

275. c) The blood flow in the injection area

276. c) To serve as a reference for doctors regarding legal medications in the US

277. c) Section 4

278. d) Intravenous (IV) administration

279. a) Patient's preference

280. c) Topical application

281. b) Cardiology

282. b) Neurologist

283. d) Internal organs

284. b) Skin, hair, and nails

285. d) Amputation

286. c) Medical geneticist

287. d) To assist with weight loss

288. b) Gastroenterologist

289. c) Treating eye conditions

290. b) Geriatric medicine

291. c) Endocrinology

292. a) Abdominoplasty

293. b) Genetic disorders

294. c) Obstetrics/gynecology

295. c) Examining tissue samples for diagnoses

296. c) Plastic surgery

297. c) Hematologist

298. c) Treating infectious diseases

299. b) Immunologist/allergist

300. b) Anesthesiology

Dear Reader,

As I pen down this note, my heart swells with gratitude. Your support means more than words can express. As a small author, every page I write is a step towards realizing my dreams, not just for myself but for my family. Each book I craft is a piece of my soul; having you journey through it is a gift I cherish.

In the vast expanse of non-fiction literature, readers like you enable authors like me to continue our pursuit of truth and understanding. But your support doesn't just touch my life. It ripple effect benefits my family, my dedicated employees, and their families. Every book you pick up contributes to sustaining our collective dreams and aspirations.

If the content of this book has resonated with you and provided value, please leave a review. Such endorsements guide fellow readers on their knowledge journey and bolster our commitment to producing impactful work. It's a small gesture, but one that has a profound impact.

Thank you for being an integral part of our shared mission. With your continued support, I am inspired to delve deeper, research more diligently, and craft content that can touch countless lives.

With profound gratitude,

Team at First Try Press

Made in the USA
Columbia, SC
13 September 2024

42241160R00143